AF070182

READING HANDS
FOR HEALTH AND HEALING

READING HANDS FOR HEALTH AND HEALING

Palm Diagnostics for Medical Conditions

Johnny Fincham

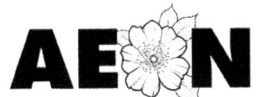

First published in 2025 by
Aeon Books Ltd

Copyright © 2025 by Johnny Fincham

The right of Johnny Fincham to be identified as the author of this work has been asserted in accordance with §§ 77 and 78 of the Copyright Design and Patents Act 1988.

All rights reserved. No part of this publication may be reproduced, stored in a retrieval system, or transmitted, in any form or by any means, electronic, mechanical, photocopying, recording, or otherwise, without the prior written permission of the publisher.

British Library Cataloguing in Publication Data

A C.I.P. for this book is available from the British Library

ISBN: 978-1-80152-165-9

Printed in Great Britain

www.aeonbooks.co.uk

*This book is dedicated to my wonderful wife, Jo Richardson,
and amazing son, Jai-Jai.
Also to my brother-in-law, Kevin Whincup,
and to all carers, healers, and therapists everywhere.*

CONTENTS

Introduction		1
1	Getting started	6
2	Constitutional types	11
3	Playing detective – taking handprints	21
4	Armour-plated or supersensitive?	25
5	The thumb and thumb ball	30
6	The fingers	36
7	Fingerprint patterns	43
8	Dermatoglyphics and disease	54
9	The major lines	61
10	The major earth line	67
11	The major air line	79
12	The water line	94
13	The fire line	108
14	Minor lines	119

15	Stress!	133
16	Skin ridge break-up, string of pearls	143
17	Involuntary hand tremors	148
18	The nails	151
19	Common acute conditions	167

APPENDIX		175
INDEX		177

READING HANDS
FOR HEALTH AND HEALING

Introduction

We live in a world obsessed with health and with maximising our physical potential. The internet provides us with millions of sites offering various diets, fitness regimes, lifestyle advice, superfood fads, well-being gurus, energy boosting tips, strategies for particular diseases, and over a thousand different therapies. More than 6.5 million health-related internet searches are placed every single day.

A 2019 survey commissioned by LetsGetChecked and conducted by OnePol found that 65% of people in the United States had tried diagnosing themselves on Google. Of those respondents, 74% said these attempts had caused them stress. And, perhaps more frighteningly, the diagnoses found online were inaccurate more than half of the time, with people falsely convincing themselves that they have serious illnesses. Despite the fact that we live in a world that is seen vast technological improvements in scanning, diagnosing, and dealing with multiple health problems, we still have a long way to go to find a simple method to spot an underlying condition before it becomes manifest.

That method is quite literally, in the palm of your hands. Your hands, in terms of their shape, appearance, skin texture, markings, fingernails, lines, and fingerprints, give an astonishingly quick and well-proven reflection of the state of your health. This is something that has been recognised since at least the time of Hippocrates – the father of modern medicine. Way back in the fifth century BC, Hippocrates described a condition called digital clubbing (a swelling, curved quality of the fingernails similar to upside-down spoons) in a patient with empyema (where pus fills the space between the lungs and the membrane around it). This is still valid as a sign of empyema today.

Aristotle, the first true scientist, Paracelsus, the creator of therapeutics, Dr Charles Bell, whose essay drawing a distinction between sensory and motor nerves is considered by many to be the founding stone of clinical neurology, all studied the human hand as a diagnostic tool. As the *Journal of the American Medical Association* (JAMA) stated in 1994:

> Despite widespread and sometimes unnecessary use of numerous laboratory tests in day-by-day practice, diagnostic methods that require no special apparatus and depend only on simple observation can play an effective role in obtaining clinical information about patients. In this connection, the human hand is a unique organ from which an extraordinary amount of clinical information may be derived.

Perhaps one of the greatest strengths of modern hand reading is that it presents an holistic, multi-layered model of an individual. This means that it is possible to read the palm as a way of illuminating the psychological, emotional, and underlying attitudes, behaviours, and states of being that cause potential illness. Modern medicine is amazing at dealing with trauma and infection. However, as the body is perceived as a mechanical system of chemical interactions, a one-dimensional approach to everything, from chronic issues like cancer to simple ones like indigestion, means that the patient is given drugs. These often come with multiple side effects that don't deal with the underlying problem. Mental health is a crucial and proven aspect of physical health. The hand reveals in great detail this dimension of the healing process – the attitudes, issues, and mindsets that caused the disease in the body, which ultimately must be remedied before proper healing can take place. Only in the holistic, emotional, and psychological dimension can we fully understand and heal the whole body–mind. Complementary therapists have long understood how fear, anger, obsession, repression, and so on drive the diseases that eventually overcome our systems. Palm reading can show us exactly the how, where, and why a medical issue has arisen and what steps need to be taken to repair and resolve the problem.

Palmistry's history is a very long one indeed, dating back to at least 2000 BC. For most of this time, it has unfortunately been burdened with an air of fatalism, fear, and superstition. Until the last quarter of the twentieth century, palmistry was primarily a form of prediction, using markings on the lines as a way of seeing (generally negative) future events. Most traditional palmists had no understanding of the fact that the lines on the palm change over time, nor that changes in the hand reflect changing attitudes, states of mind, and health patterns. Only fairly recently, in 1936, did this view begin to change, when the physician and psychoanalyst Charlotte Wolff identified distinct palm patterns of those with severe learning disorders. As a trained hand reader and physician working in a series of mental hospitals, she was able to demonstrate clear and obvious differences in the palms of those born with congenital illnesses and to identify particular conditions from the hands. This provided a starting point for serious investigation into the hands as way of predicting personality, genetic illnesses, as well as possible disease. A huge amount of research was begun in the 1980s into the links between fingerprint patterns and a disposition to particular health issues. In very recent times, the anthropological researcher John Manning has conducted experiments proving that certain finger-length configurations indicate definite human characteristics, with important health correspondences. Well over 8,000 research papers have been published in the last five decades on links between the palm and disease.

Considering the fact that one third of the brain's motor and sensory cortex is devoted to the palms, it is not difficult to establish the connection between what is happening in the hand and what is going on in the mind. (See Figure I.1.)

The palm provides a unique window into the inner workings of an individual's mind state. We can easily illustrate the link between brain development and hand development with a condition like, for instance, Down's syndrome. The differences between Down's

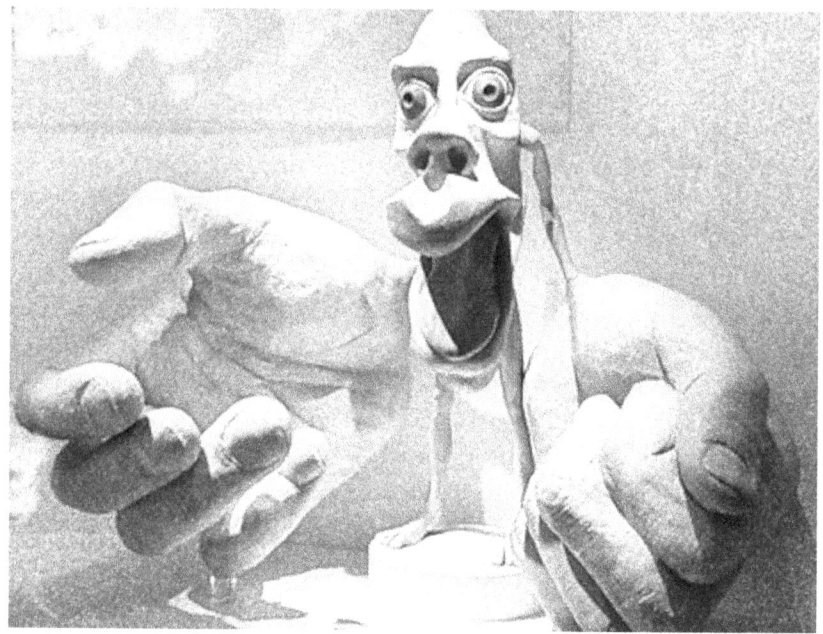

Figure I.1. The body in proportion to brain motor and nerve allocation.

syndrome hands and so-called normals has been recognised for over a century. The hands in Down's have an easily discernible set of characteristics that are very obvious – a small, square palm with short fingers; the palm has only a few crudely marked lines, and the two transverse creases (traditionally called the heart line and the head line) are combined into one single line (called a single transverse palmar crease – STPC). The single transverse crease is often known (in a somewhat prejudiced manner) as the simian line. In Down's, the single crease is accompanied by a short, bent, or deformed little finger, and all digits have low-lying loop patterns on them. (See Figure I.2.)

This should convince anyone that the hand is a window onto the development of mind, personality, and character. The rich and fascinating story of medical palmistry is still being written, and the study of this amazing process will give you not only insights into the state of anyone's health, but a deep look into their psycho-

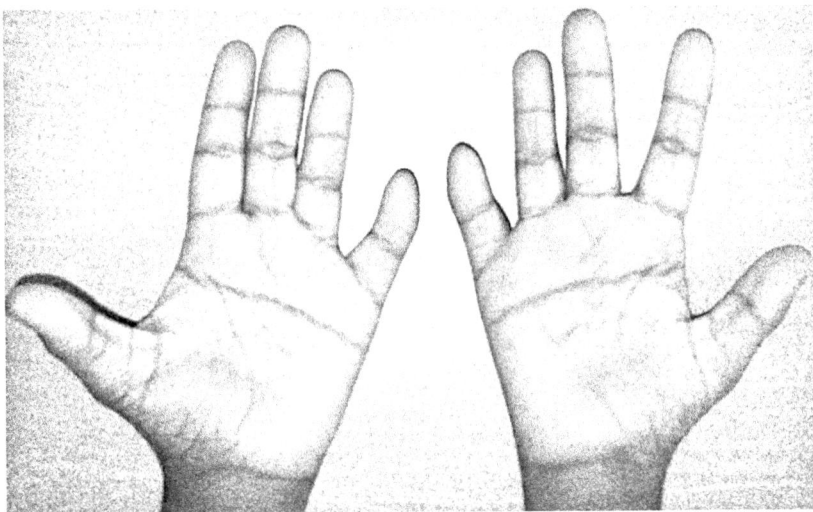

Figure I.2. Down's syndrome hand.

logical, mental, and emotional nature – a multi-level hologram of the human being.

Sources

Hert, M. de, et al. "Physical illness in patients with severe mental disorders." *World Psychiatry*, Vol. 10, No. 1 (2011): 52–77.

JAMA. "The hand and cardiovascular disease." *Journal of the American Medical Association*, Vol. 154, No. 6 (1994): 508.

LetsGetChecked survey by OnePoll. "Two in five people misdiagnosed themselves with "serious diseases" after consulting "Dr Google'". *Daily Mail*, 8 November 2019. https://www.dailymail.co.uk/health/article-7666059/2-5-people-misdiagnosed-consulting-Dr-Google.html

Manning, J. *The Finger Book* (London: Faber & Faber, 2009).

MIND. *Mental Health Facts and Statistics Report, 2023*. https://www.mind.org.uk/information-support/types-of-mental-health-problems/mental-health-facts-and-statistics

Wolff, C. *The Human Hand* (Methuen, 1942).

1

Getting started

First of all, we should start with a warning. If you are a palm reader, it's vital to recognise that you aren't medically qualified, so don't diagnose – ever. Even if you're absolutely sure you've seen the signs of a serious disease on someone's palm, only advise that they have a check-up with a professional as soon as possible. Medicine is a vast, complex, hugely specialised area. There are over 300 types of cancer, for instance, and 63 different blood disorders, so we cannot, as hand readers, possibly claim to be able to specify exactly what condition or illness a person is suffering from. Acquiring the ability from this book to see health conditions in the hands will not give you medical expertise. We can often quickly identify potential illness and latent issues a long time before they become chronic – as you will see, the hand is amazing at indicating disease in its early stages – but we are not going to be able to diagnose with 100% certainty. We can only point out a likely problem and urge a client to have a specialist screening. The hand presents a wonderful window into the issues that underlie a health problem, and, by advising a change of behaviour, we can often head off an illness before it becomes more serious. Big pharma and modern medicine is only really interested in dealing with a disease after it has manifested itself – usually in the form of an operation or by taking powerful pharmaceutical drugs. This is where complementary medicine can play a huge part in working with the individual when a pattern is picked up before it becomes chronic. So often, by using subtle techniques, like psychotherapy, herbs, Traditional Chinese Medicine, or massage, the client can have a condition seen in the hand treated holistically without ever going near a regular GP. The minor lines of the hand in particular can change very quickly when we alter our diets and behaviour, and signs of health problems often vanish, given the right conditions. However, we must never forget that we are looking to identify the area of the body, the deep behavioural patterns, the areas of stress or imbalance that are behind any illness, but we are not ever able to diagnose with certainty the exact nature of the disease itself.

We can cause enormous harm if we say anything to worry or distress a person whose hand we are reading. As mentioned earlier, palmistry carries a big burden of superstition and fatalism along with it, and this can easily frighten and disturb anyone who has a fear of some latent illness (which most of us have). This book is a wonderful aid to anyone who is interested in health in a wider sense, and in particular to alternative and complementary health practitioners who would like a fast, reliable, accurate method of knowing where to focus a therapy, remedy, practice, or treatment. However, proceed with caution, and always push your client towards an expert if you suspect any condition.

In this book we look at the hand as a diagnostic tool from a series of frames, from the overall constitutional types, through various markers and signs that point to genetic likelihood of a disease, and slowly work through to more specific indicators of a medical conditions being currently present. Ideally, there should be three signs of any condition for you to be sure of an illness or issue, and even then, however convinced you are of a problem you must gently persuade your client towards an expert, a therapist, a second opinion, or a thorough examination, without pronouncing your verdict. The mind has powers that are deeper and more powerful than we are yet aware of, and fear and stress can do much harm. So proceed gently and guide, rather than diagnose.

Active and passive hands

In palmistry the dominant hand is known as the active hand; the other is the passive. For most people (90% of the population) the right hand is the dominant hand and is used for writing or catching a ball. The passive hand is controlled by the intuitive, emotion-ruled hemisphere of the brain, and the dominant palm is controlled by the rational and logical hemisphere. The passive hand reflects the passive, internalised, more subliminal, buried, child-like part of our personality. The active hand reveals our more developed, public, active, conscious and focused personality. The passive hand is much more representative of how we are as raw, unprocessed, child-like beings. Health and psychological issues that have been imprinted, inherited, or triggered in childhood are likely to be seen here. Often behaviours, attitudes, and programmes passed down from generations back in the family are seen in the passive hand. Only our parents and those intimate with us would know us as the person presented in the passive hand.

Both hands are always taken into account in a reading. Usually, the passive hand has more markings, the lines are more fragmented and more poorly formed. An active hand that has stronger, clearer lines indicates that health and general psychology is greatly improved as a person has matured and grown to adulthood. However, if the patterns in the lines appear worse, more broken up, and messy in the active hand, it's likely that an inherited physical or mental health issue is a long-term pre-existing condition and has become more pronounced as time has gone on. The passive hand will tell us about our inherited predispositions to disease – what could happen if we were to abuse our systems. The markings in our active or dominant hands show the sort of illnesses that are likely to become manifest.

GETTING STARTED 9

Time and tide

One of the greatest myths perpetuated by old fashioned predictive palmists is that the lines of the palm are fixed and show one's "destiny". A quick look at the handprints of the same person a few years apart will quickly dispense with this idea. As can be seen in Figure 1.1, the lines and markings on this palm have changed significantly.

As we evolve, grow, and particularly as we develop or heal from physical and psychological conditions, the hands reflect these changes. Children's hand's in particular show changes rapidly as they grow (Figures 1.2).

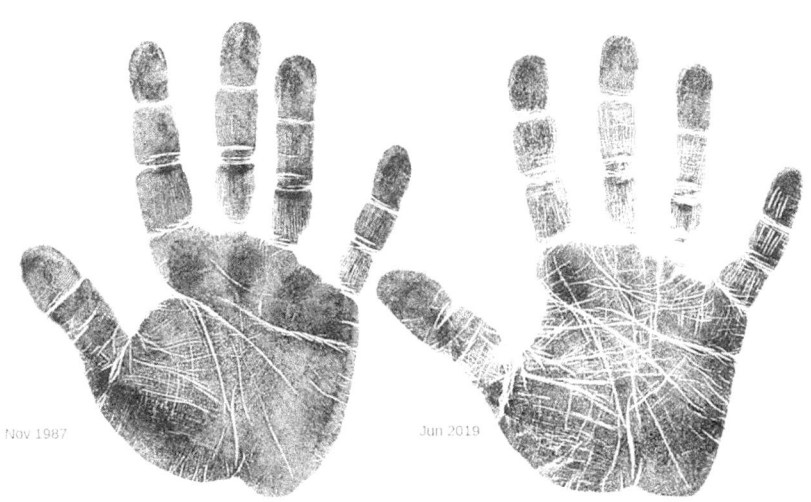

Figure 1.1. Changed hands.

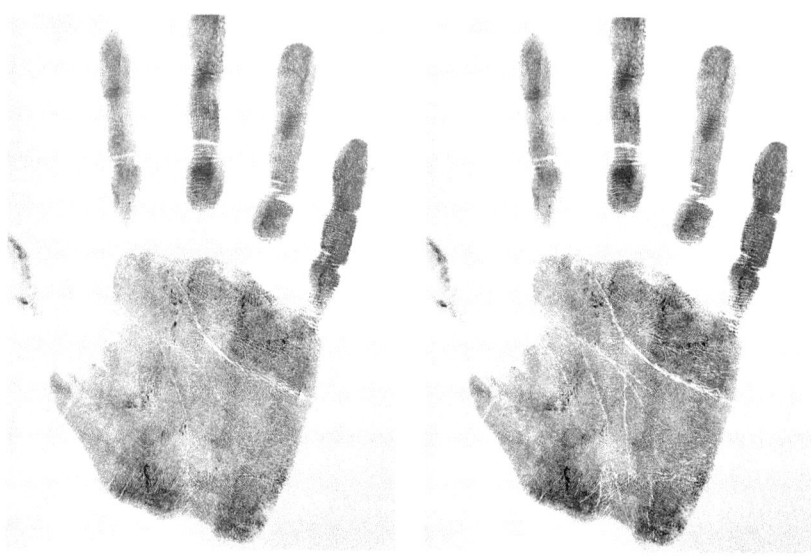

Figure 1.2 (*Left*) Six-year-old child's hand. (*Right*) Same child seven months later.

2

Constitutional types

We'll start our study with a look at basic constitutions. In palmistry, there are four fundamental hand shapes that correspond to four basic constitutions, character types, and physical natures. Each of these four types, with a different nature, physical strength and weakness, and approach to life corresponds to one the four elements of fire, water, earth, and air. This does not mean by any means that a disorder or disease is present in any type of hand, but it gives us a starting point for atypical disease patterns that are likely to emerge in these four genetic types.

The idea that these four elements – earth, water, air, and fire – made up all matter was the cornerstone of philosophy, science, and medicine for two thousand years. The four elements are used in many traditional medicinal and spiritual systems, including astrology, paganism, design, art, and Hindu and Buddhist cosmology. An understanding of the elements is a key to perceiving human nature, the energies that move within and around us, and how the world works in a profound, spiritual way. Each of the element character types has inherent strengths and weaknesses.

Judging the elemental nature of a hand is the first step in how we ascertain the constitution, nature, and areas of the body where problems are likely to occur. Knowing the four hand and body types makes a nonsense of the endless over-promoted diets and supplements that come and go as fashion dictates. We need to shape our health habits and nutrition around our individual constitutions – "one man's meat is another man's poison" is an old but very true adage.

The four palm shape patterns are: square palms with short fingers: earth hands; square palms with long fingers: air hands; rectangular palms with short fingers: fire hands; and narrow rectangular palms with long fingers: water hands. The elemental palm shapes are shown in Figure 2.1.

When you examine a hand looking for the element, remember that hands must be judged loosely, as a palm is never exactly square or precisely rectangular; flesh and blood are not geometrical straight edges and angles. If the fingers are spread out, it can make it difficult to decide if the fingers are long or not. Try to judge the palm shape with the fingers closed together. You are judging the overall form, look, and sense of the palm. The four palm shapes reflect their respective elements not just in shape, but in their *feel* as well. Earth palms give a sense of weight: the hands feel heavy, with thick bones that give a still, solid quality. Water palms feel pliant and loose: they have a refined, soft, gentle sense. Fire palms are hot and muscular, the palm is vibrant and restless. Air hands give a spacious energy: they are the biggest palms, but are light-boned and bird-like.

Some people (around a quarter of the population) have undefined palms, with rounded sides and mid-length fingers, where the elements are mixed and the hands are difficult to categorise. In this case, simply ignore the hand shape altogether.

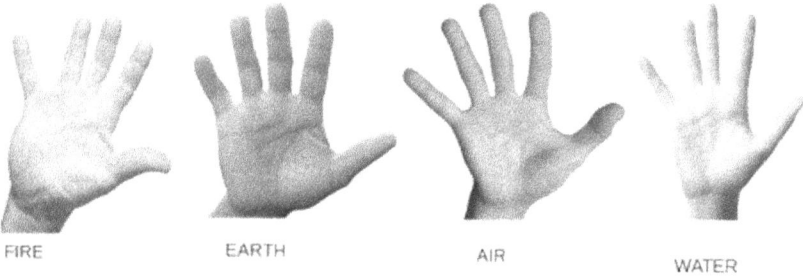

FIRE   EARTH   AIR   WATER

Figure 2.1. The four elemental hand shapes.

The earth element

The palms of earth people (Figure 2.2) are thicker, heavier, and more fleshy than the other hand types. The palm is square, with fingers that are short, denoting the primal demands of the palm dominating the intellectual qualities of the fingers. Earth hands have gravity and weight, the bones are thick and strong, the mounts well formed and solid, the lines deep and strong.

Physically, earth types tend to be short, with thick, strong bones and strong teeth; they have a sense of physical presence. They are innately robust, and they like to live physical lives, tending to have lots of pets and children. There is always a preference for a rural, simple life over one that is city-based, cosmopolitan and stressful. As they are born with resilient constitutions, they have deep resources of endurance and stamina. Their body is naturally strong, with large muscles, and they tend to move slowly, hating

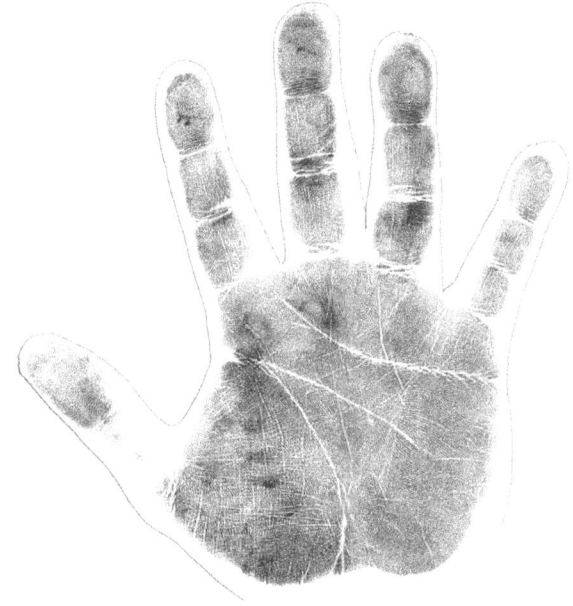

Figure 2.2.   Earth hand.

to rush. Earth types are out of tune with the current trend for stick-thin bodies; they often force their broad profiles into diet regimes, and for them this is potentially harmful. It is essential that they learn to love the strength, power, and stamina their solid physicality endows them with. A certain physical broadness is their norm.

Common health problems of an earth nature are failing to keep moving and using their bodies enough, so they can easily slip into obesity and diseases of stagnation, as they love their food. A mainly vegetarian diet with lots of grains, seeds, and nuts is ideal. Their dogged, habitual nature tends to get fixed in patterns, so they can obstinately eat traditional, unhealthy foods and find it hard to change. They can be excessively fatalistic about life expectancy and health outcomes. Earth types naturally repress emotions and tend to hold on to past grievances. Stomach and digestive issues, constipation, and high cholesterol, as well as hip- and lower spine degeneration are classic earth hand health problems.

By nature, earth hands have the best health, but they all too often ignore problems, leave them to fate or the "experts", and let nature take its course. They can all too readily accept illness and old age. For earth types it's essential to avoid modern, fast, stressful lifestyles. They must get lots of fresh air and get outdoors. They must not allow themselves to get into unhealthy ruts; they need to maintain steady routines, habits, and life patterns that keep them mobile, grounded, and stable.

Always check the condition of the earth line (to be studied later in this book), as an earth hand with a weak earth line is like a castle with weak foundations.

The water element

The water hand (Figure 2.3) has long, dreamy fingers, with narrow palms. The skin on the hands has numerous fine lines and the digits are very flexible, denoting fluid mental processes. Water-handed people are loose, pliable, changeable, moody, emotionally

CONSTITUTIONAL TYPES 15

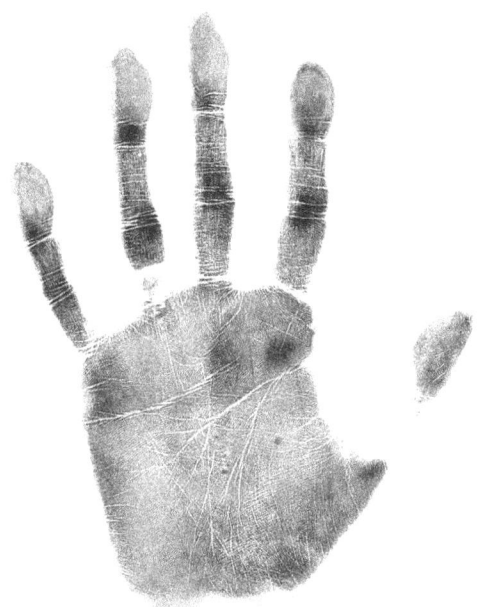

Figure 2.3. Water hand.

driven, and very affected by the people and situations around them. Invariably – whether male or female – they have long hair. Usually pale-skinned, they tend to have bodies that are soft and plump or willowy and slender.

The water type has the weakest constitution. Highly adaptable, they often bend too far in caring and responding to others. They suffer from immune-system disorders, breast cancer, gynaecological and prostate problems, prolapsed organs and muscles, weakness of the lower back (lordosis), kidney complaints, over-extension of the joints, and connective tissue problems. Water types are suited to any vocation that involves people and children, the caring, social professions, alternative and complementary forms of healthcare, massage, mysticism, spiritual development, fantasy, and the arts. The water type needs to avoid driven, competitive financial- and goal-orientated situations – they need peace and harmony in their surroundings. Relationships are a particular danger area, as they can turn in on themselves and become unstable when relationships go wrong. Water-handed people need good-quality cold pressed oils, soups and stews, smoothies, tofu, seafood, easy-to-digest diets and lots of fresh green leafy vegetables and salads.

Always check the water line when you find a water hand. A problem with the water line on a water hand is like finding a fish that struggles to swim.

The fire element

The fire hand (Figure 2.4) is rectangular, but wider than a water palm, so there is a degree of adaptability, and the digits are quite short, but they are not so short as an earth hand's fingers. The digits are stiff and often knotty. Fire hands are almost always warm, giving off an aura of heat and movement. The skin is usually grainy and the lines on the palm are deep and red, like cuts.

In terms of body type, the fire body is slightly short, with well-developed muscularity – the body usually tanned or adorned with tattoos and piercings. Usually, whether male or female the hair is short, functional and out of the way and the eyes have a direct, intense quality.

The fire mindset denoted is not academic, but able to synthesise information quickly and therefore sees the whole picture but has little time for details. Fire types prefer to act rather than deliberate as they have little patience for those slower than themselves. They are liable to take things to extremes as they are highly competitive. Fire types are always pursuing goals and seek to attain more power and status by hard work and relentless drive. Fire types are the most likely to have plastic surgery or to develop an ideal physique. They need a lot of high-quality protein, beans, pulses, the minerals, iron and magnesium and to avoid strongly spiced, hot foods.

In terms of health, the fire type is prone to overwork, and as they find it hard to relax and can be guilty of using various narcotics, legal and illegal, either to get more energy or to calm themselves down. Fire people are prone to burn out, alcoholism,

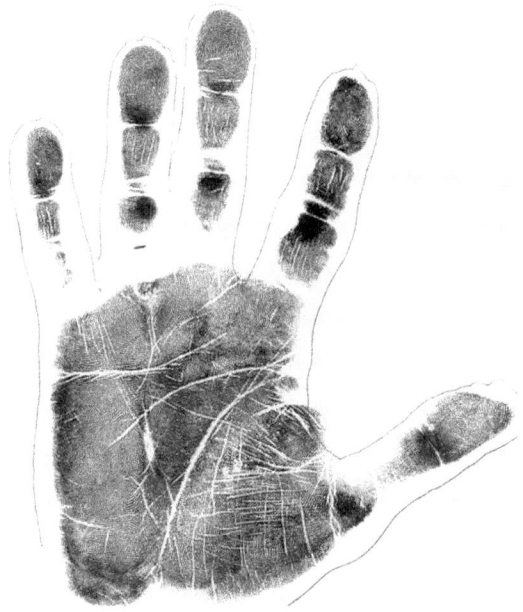

Figure 2.4. Fire hand.

addictions, heart attacks, stomach ulcers, heartburn, excess acidity, accidents and muscle strain, injury, car accidents and broken bones. As the fire person has no natural capacity to relax, they need a lively form of switching off and calming down: dancing, aerobics, fitness classes, surfing and skiing are classic fire activities.

Check the fire line on any fire hand. A fire hand with a poor or missing fire line is like a racing car with no steering wheel.

The air element

The hand of air types (Figure 2.5) is large and square in shape, giving a rational, material framework to their natures; they have the longest fingers, denoting their intellectual approach to life.

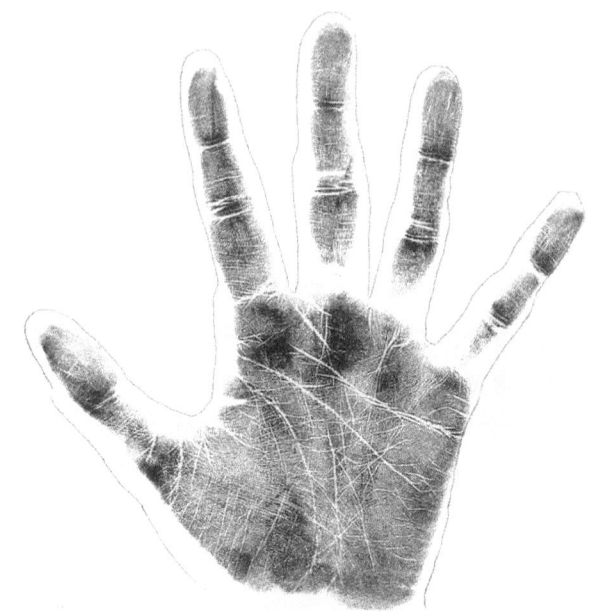

Figure 2.5. Air palm.

The finger bones are light, thin, and bird-like, and the skin is dry, yellowish, and papery, with long, fine lines. The air type tends to be tall and naturally thin, with fine, sparse hair; they are light-boned and have an elevated air about them.

Air people love to study, teach, communicate, and learn. They are eccentric, aloof, thoughtful, studious, and their minds are a blizzard of ideas. The classic air archetype is the bespectacled university lecturer or nerdy computer scientist or a specialist of some kind, whose knowledge gives them authority. Air people are inclined to put principle before practicality and often fail to follow through on projects at ground level. Air types need to eat regular small meals as their digestive capacity is limited. They can easily to forget to eat, digesting big ideas instead. They must avoid drinking too much tea and coffee and snacking on junk foods and foods with a high sugar content.

Classic health issues with the air type are short-sightedness and eye problems, nervous complaints, anxiety, upper back and neck problems, and also breathing, lungs, and skin issues.

It is important for the air type to avoid stress and to keep a good connection to the body and to avoid faddish diets, inconstant routines, and overthinking.

Good practice is to do sports that require speed and timing, like running, cycling, badminton, and squash, at which they naturally excel.

Examine the air line on any air palm. A poor air line on an air hand is like a bird that cannot fly.

Undefined palms

No clear elemental hand shape? No problem!

If a person has a hand shape that doesn't conform to an element, this is actually a good thing. The palm might bulge in the middle and have a rounded quality to the sides, so it's not rectangular or square, or it might be broader at the base than the area near the fingers. There could also be fingers of middling length, neither long nor short, and the palm neither hot, cool, light, or heavy. This is a mixed hand, and genetically this shows a kind of combination of various elemental and ancestral types that typically give a broad spectrum of immune diversity and latent strengths, so they are less likely to have inherent weaknesses. A quarter of people have mixed-element hands. If you see the pure elemental hands as kind of thoroughbreds with specific strengths and built-in weaknesses in terms of health issues, the mixed hand is a kind of mongrel or mixed breed that has the best of all strengths but few inherent vulnerabilities.

As the palm in Figure 2.6 is slightly triangular, it's difficult to discern the shape.

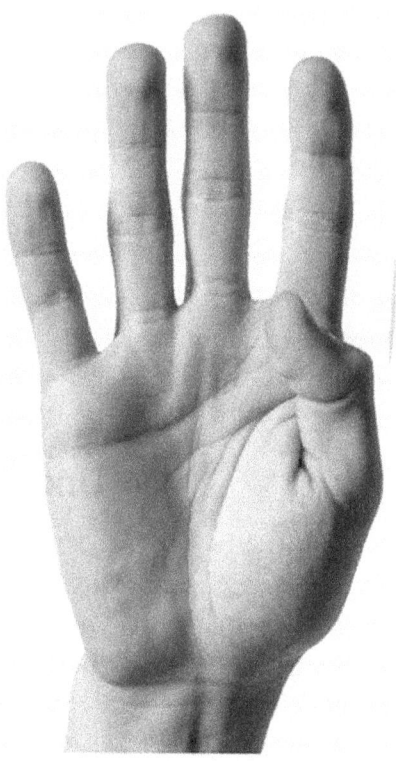

Figure 2.6. Mixed palm.

3

Playing detective – taking handprints

In order to examine the finer points of medical palm reading, we need to take handprints to capture the details of skin ridge patterns and to see markings invisible to the naked eye. As you investigate prints of hands, you will see all sorts of details – skin ridge patterns, fingerprint formations, fine lines, islands, and minor markings that are not possible to see without an imprint of the hand. Using a magnifying glass and taking prints of a palm at regular intervals will allow you to observe changes that occur as people adapt to different life choices and health programmes. It is very rewarding to watch as broken skin ridges heal, lines become clearer, and negative markings vanish when nutrition and balanced lifestyles are adapted.

Method

You will need block printing, water-based ink in black or a dark colour, an ink roller around 10 cm long (both available from arts and crafts shops), and plain A4 photocopying paper. (See Figure 3.1)

1. Squeeze a pea-sized blob of ink onto any smooth non-absorbent surface like a magazine with a glossy cover. Roll the ink with the roller until you have a patch of ink about a foot square and the roller is covered in a thin layer all over, from edge to edge. Try to use the very minimum amount of ink possible, as too much will result in a blotchy print.
2. Roll the ink carefully all over the palm, covering the whole surface including the fingers and fingertips with an even,

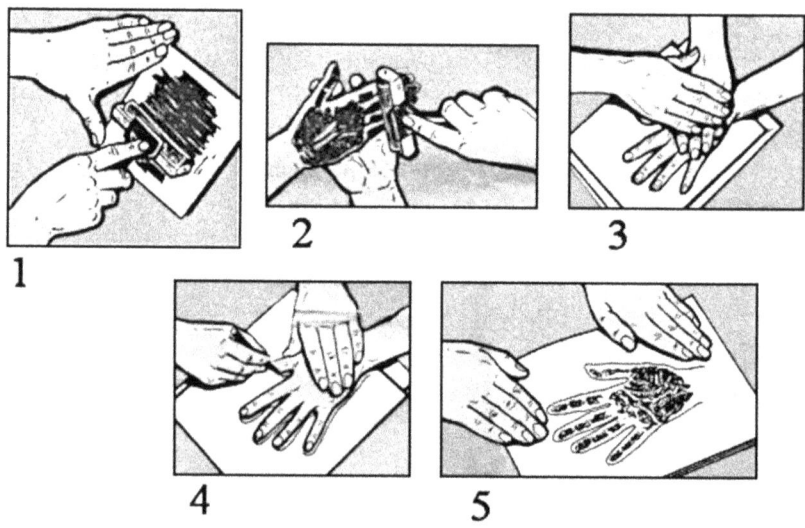

Figure 3.1. Taking palm prints.

fine layer. Those having their print taken tend to stretch out their palm while the ink is applied, but this makes the lines more sharply defined than they naturally are, so it's best to get them to relax their hands as much as possible. Follow the contours of the hand, and dab the roller onto any bare patches, using it like a paintbrush.
3. Place a couple of magazines under some plain A4 paper. Then press the client's inked palm down onto the paper with firm pressure, using both your own hands. Do this quickly before the ink starts to dry out. Make sure you push down on the whole of the palm and fingers, so all of the inner hand makes contact with the paper.
4. Draw around the palm and fingers, as this gives you a better idea of the outline and elemental shape of the palm. Then lift the hand off carefully, holding the printed paper down with one hand while you do so.
5. Write the person's name and age on the paper. Then there is a shorthand you can use to indicate various qualities of the palm that cannot be ascertained from a print alone. You will learn these qualities in later chapters, and you will need these details for future reference. Handedness is illustrated with RHA for right-handed and LHA for a left-handed person. Stiffness of the fingers and thumbs is indicated by a number, where 5 is floppy, 3 is average, and 1 is rigidly immobile. The thumb's print pattern won't normally come out, as the thumb is naturally held side on to the paper. Once you've learned the various print formations, write down the print pattern on the thumbs. Also, write down whether the Venus mount is particularly soft or large and well formed.

When reading palms, the need for good light cannot be overemphasised. An illuminated magnifying glass is extremely useful; it doesn't need to be of particularly high magnification.

The finished print should look something like Figure 3.2.

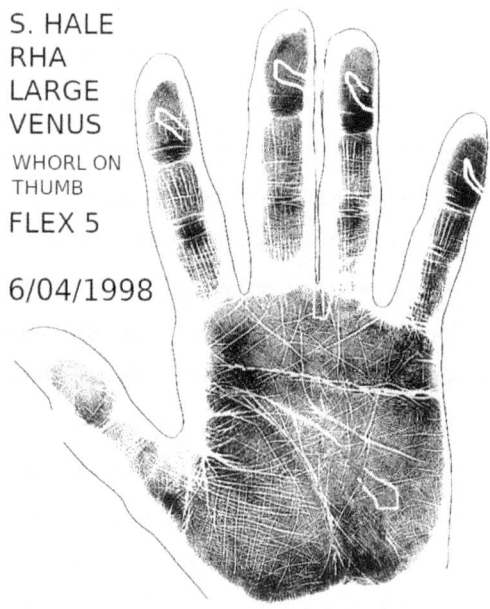

Figure 3.2. Palm print.

4

Armour-plated or supersensitive?

A crucial health issue is a persons' overall sensitivity, and this is indicated by the skin texture on the inside of the palm.

Skin texture

The skin on the inner palm is of vital importance. It indicates the physical responsiveness of a person and how they react to the world around them (Figure 4.1). The quality of the skin texture on the inside of the palm is a guide to how complex and responsive the central nervous system is. Research has shown that the greater the number of nerve connections to the brain from the hand's skin surface, the greater the intricacy of the nervous system as a whole (Department of Scientific and Industrial Research, New Zealand). The skin on the inner palm is covered in very fine, raised dermal ridges, with multiple sweat glands and nerve receptors embedded in them. These receptors can detect heat, cold, pain, pressure, vibrations, feel, and texture, and in very fine skin

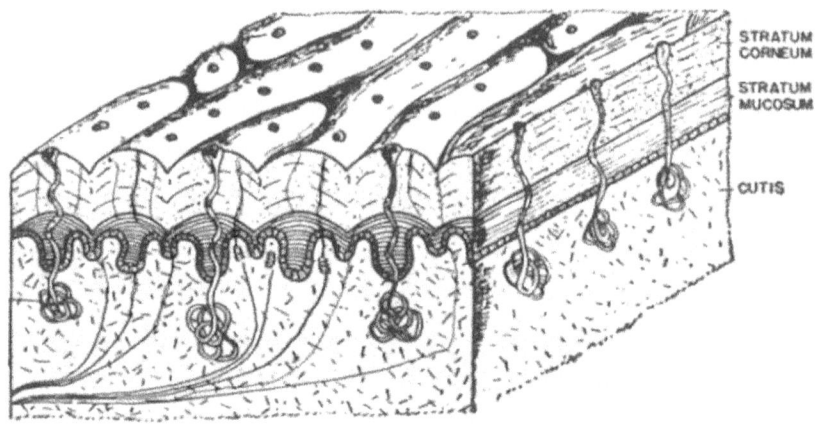

Figure 4.1. Cross-section of the ridges in palmar skin.

they detect subtle energies and atmospheres that the majority of us are unaware of.

The skin on the inside of the palm varies from person to person in thickness and how complex and dense the dermal ridges are. These ridges cover the whole inner palm and fingertips and form the fingerprints. Most palms tend to have skin that varies between the feel of soft paper and that of leather (men tend to have coarser palm skin than females). Some individuals, however, have exceptionally delicate, complex, and super-fine skin, and some rare individuals have very rough, coarse skin, almost like wood. Both these skin types have huge health implications.

There are two ways to check skin texture: you can simply feel the surface using the tip of your index finger, stroking it across the middle of the palm (or an area near the centre where there are no calluses). A second method also is to look at the print of a palm and examine the skin ridges and the number, density, and quality of the lines present.

Thin skin

If you feel thin, silky palmar skin with multiple, closely packed skin ridges that gives easily under your fingertip (Figure 4.2), this flags up the classic supersensitive soul. It is immediately obvious when you run your finger over the inside of the palm – you won't be able to feel the skin ridges at all. The skin feels ultra-soft and smooth, and the palm print always shows a multiple of fine, scratchy lines all over. This skin quality affects everything about a person, including their diet, career, lifestyle, habits, and the type of relationships they can have. This high level of sensitivity indicates a person easily overwhelmed in reaction to their environment. Super-sensitives must be careful not to expose themselves to the toxins and tensions of modern life. Car fumes, dust, bedbugs, cigarette smoke, stressful atmospheres, electrical fields, recreational substances like coffee, alcohol, over-the-counter medicines, additives in foods, highly spiced meals, etc., can all cause the system to overload. This skin type creates a fussy, fragile disposition and someone who is hyper-aware of hot and cold, atmospheres, stress, and bad energy. Hypersensitives find they cannot tolerate an adult dose of many medicines, and they are highly responsive to subtle therapies, like homeopathy, spiritual healing, and reiki. It is strongly recommended to advise those with this type of heightened sensitivity to use their awareness in a positive manner by working in the fields of complementary therapies, in spiritual, intuitive, and mystical realms, and also in the arts, where being highly aware is a valuable asset. They must at all costs maintain a clean diet and a lifestyle that allows them to avoid the toxins and tensions of modern life.

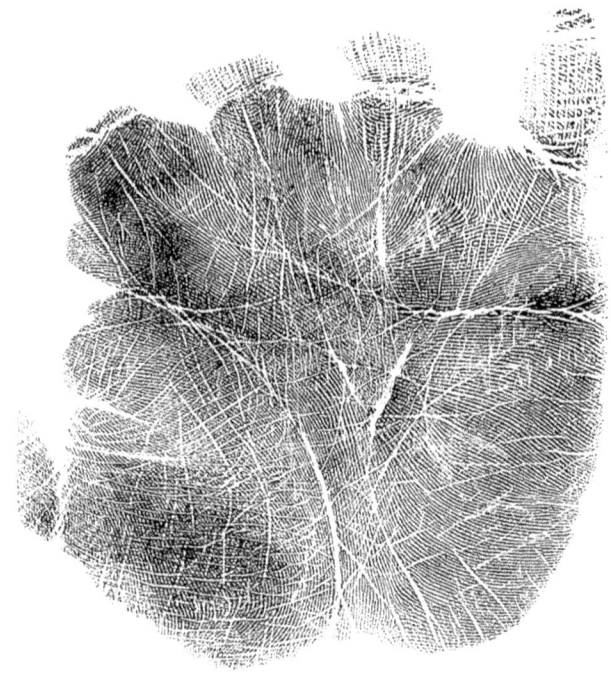

Figure 4.2. Silk skin.

Coarse skin

The other extreme of skin (and of awareness and sensitivity) is ultra-coarse skin (Figure 4.3). This will only be found on hardy outdoor types who are impervious to the weather, heavy physical work, pain, and temperature. Coarse skin is found almost exclusively on males, and they are the very last type to seek any kind of medical support. Coarse skin can easily be seen by examining the lines of the hand, which are few in number (often only three or four lines are present), and the lines are very thick and trough like. If you brush your fingertip over the inside of the palm, it feels hard and rough, like old shoe leather. Coarse-skinned people are

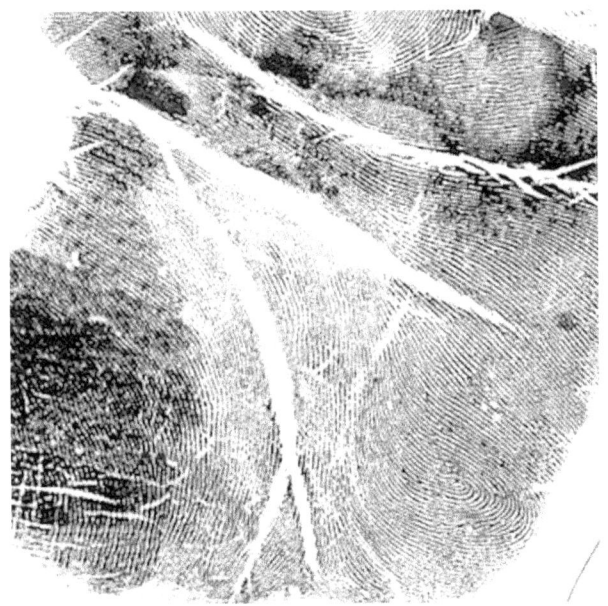

Figure 4.3. Coarse skin.

very prone to accidents, industrial diseases, dust inhalation, injury, neglect, infections, and joint issues. As they are extremely robust and unaffected by physical hardships, they tend to disregard all health advice, trusting that their strong natures will prevail, and they tend to scoff at alternative medicine and dietary guidelines. All too often their self-neglect and taste for "heavy fuel" fry ups, pies, cakes, junk food, and so on will eventually cause their systems to break down.

Source

Department of Scientific and Industrial Research, New Zealand. *Skin Texture on Inner Palms and Neurological Complexity.* Unpublished paper, No. 5569-0113, 27 May 1998.

5

The thumb and thumb ball

Control, willpower, and resources

In palmistry, the thumb is the vital indicator of willpower, grip, and self-discipline. The thumb is the key to human evolution as a species, because the oppositional thumb gave us the ability to form a gripping motion. From this, humanoids developed the ability to make tools and become dominant over other species, with the use of hand-formed flints, weapons, and hunting technology. The thumb and the thumb ball muscle have grown massively in proportion to the rest of the hand over aeons as we developed from primates to modern humans. Other primates, like orangutans, have only a tiny, rudimentary thumb. "Had it not been for the unique manner of the thumb's development, humanity as we know it would not have evolved, and that colossal jump from holding and throwing stones to manufacturing interstellar spacecraft could never have been made" (David Brandon-Jones, "Physiognomy of the Hand") .

The thumb and thumb ball are important in medical analysis, because it's a measure of the innate vitality, energy store, and "grip" a person has on themselves and on life.

A good metaphor to use for the thumb is that of a rudder, holding a person to their aims and steering them to fulfilling their full potential. The thumb ball is the engine that gives the power and vitality to push a person into life. A strong, stiff thumb with a large, full thumb ball is like a big engine and a strong rudder that drives a soul onward, confronting life's challenges head on. If a person's thumb is floppy and weak and the thumb ball is flat and flabby, it's foolish to put them on a 10-day fast, for example, as the will and drive are not available. The thumb and thumb ball can be made stronger through deliberate effort, but it will need to be built up with gentle encouragement, on a slow incline, and with lots of support.

The first quality to check is the stiffness of the thumb. All children tend to have loose thumbs, so this is relevant only after the age of 17 or so years. Thumb stiffness is measured by simply gripping a person's thumb and pulling it back towards the wrist gently. The average thumb will only move a couple of centimetres or so. A rigid-thumbed person, where there is no movement at all, applies themselves rigidly to life and pushes themselves hard. Burnout is always a possibility, especially if the thumb ball is flat. However, rigid-thumbed people can stick to strict health regimes and Spartan diets with great enthusiasm, and they put great effort into all they do.

If the thumb is floppy and bends back easily, the person is somewhat childlike and easy-going: people who smell the roses on the journey of life. This more laid-back, spontaneous type of thumb is very common on musicians, entertainers, actors, and "people-people". They need variety, fun, and stimulus to inspire them to exert themselves. It indicates someone who won't drive themselves too hard and will enjoy life's journey; it can be a healthy indication as far as stress is concerned, as long as their relaxed attitude doesn't go too far down the road of over-indulgence.

Where the thumb is extremely floppy at the base, so that it can bend back almost to the wrist, this is known as hyper-flexive. People are often proud of their hyper-flexible thumbs. However, this amount of movement signals an over-adaptable nature, someone lacking staying power and who needs constant change and stimulation. It is a bonus for an actor, for example, where one has to constantly adapt to new roles and one is driven by the demands of script or director – but they can "bend over backwards" for others and be far too accommodating. Much time and energy is spent appeasing others. Usually, hyperflexive thumbs have a need for freedom in everything and hate regimentation. Any health or exercise programme must be pleasurable and fun, with lots of rewards and encouragement, otherwise it will soon be abandoned. Incidentally, hyperflexive thumbs and fingers are a sign of the early onset of joint and ligament problems, particularly in the spine. We tend to develop more self-restraint as we mature into adults, so consequently the active hand almost always has the stiffer thumb – if this is not the case (very rare), the person has grown into a more relaxed, less disciplined person as they've matured.

Thumb angle

The angle that the thumb is naturally held can be a clue to introversion. An adult who holds their thumb permanently in a clenched fist is manifesting a retrogression to childhood or a state of anxiety, insecurity, and self-doubt. They are introverted, cautious, self-conscious, and secretive; consequently, they are often "bottled up" emotionally.

The opposite pattern, when the thumb is naturally held stretched far out from the hand, forming a right angle with the index finger, shows self-assuredness (Figure 5.1). The more the thumb is held away from the index finger, the more that individual shows extroversion, strength and self-confidence.

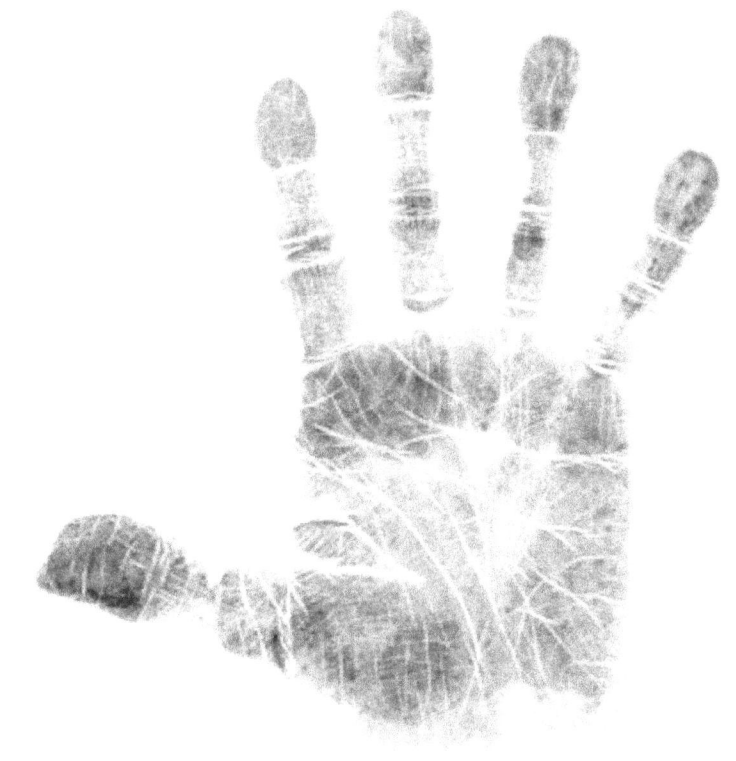

Figure 5.1.   Wide-spaced thumb.

Mount of Venus – the engine

The large, fleshy mound at the thumb's base protects the major veins and nerves that connect the hand to the rest of the body; it is known in palmistry as the Venus mount and medically as the thenar eminence. Its size and firmness is a general indicator of lust for life, capacity for human warmth, and physical resources. This is the engine that gives the thumb its grip and represents a power pack of stored drive and capacity to live fully and physically.

You can easily check this mount by pushing your own thumb strongly down into the central area of the mount itself. If your thumb pushes down easily, so you can feel the bone beneath, this is a flabby, flat mount. If there is some resistance, but there is a distinct sense of padding there and your thumb sinks in a centimetre or so, this is a good average. If your thumb barely makes an impact on the mount, if it's full and solid, this is very obvious and is the classic "power pack" mount. This indicates a person with a great energy, capacity to enjoy themselves and they will be vigorous, warm, physical and energetic. An enlarged Venus mount indicates the need to really embrace life in a full and lusty manner. Athletes, professional dancers and performers always have a large mount here (Figure 5.2).

If this mound is soft, flat, and spongy, there is a certain lassitude present – the person can lack energy and vitality. This mount will develop as the subject develops muscularity – for example, by going to the gym regularly.

The thenar eminence has been proven to deflate slowly with the ageing process. Muscle loss is a part of getting older, though not inevitably so. In a series of tests on the thumb's grip to measure

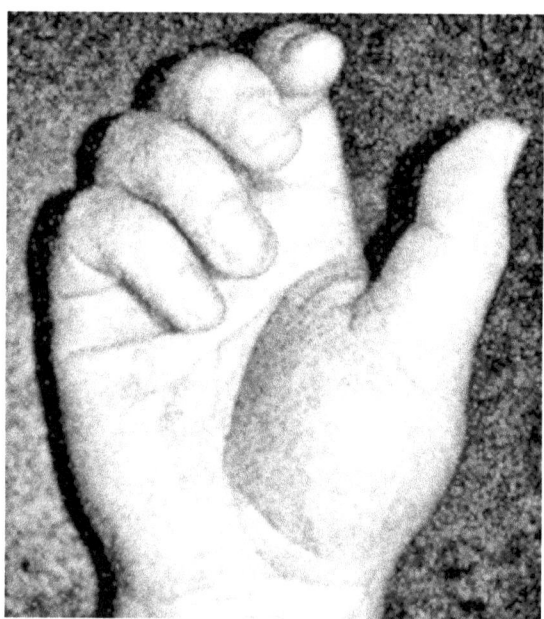

Figure 5.2. Large Venus mount on a professional footballer.

the strength of the thenar eminence muscle, scientists found that a flat, weak mount suggests poorer health outcomes generally, in particular heart health and vulnerability to various forms of cancers (Bim et al., "Handgrip Strength").

It is vital to encourage muscle development via exercise as one ages, as this prevents this mount shrinking and can even enlarge to a greater extent in old age if the exercise is programmed and progressive.

Sources

Bim, M. A., et al. "Handgrip strength and associated factors among Brazilian adolescents: A cross-sectional study." *Journal of Bodywork and Movement,* Vol. 28 (2021): 75–81.

Brandon-Jones, D. "Physiognomy of the hand." In: *Practical Palmistry* (London: Rider, 1981).

6

The fingers

The fingers deliver a rich source of information on psychological and physical health. The stiffness, comparative length, and phalange size of the digits are very rewarding to examine. In a later module, the print patterns on the fingers feed us with more health data.

Very crudely, the index, middle, ring, and little (pinky) fingers are about self, society, status, and speech. The metaphorical names we use for them are the mirror of self-reflection (index), wall of conformism (middle), peacock of self-expression (ring), and antenna of communication (little finger).

Where the body of the palm represents the primal, instinctive brain, the fingers indicate the modern, highly developed parts of the brain for ego, persona, status, conformity, communication, and other qualities that give us the ability to function in modern, complex societies.

The finger's relative growth and development is dependent on hormonal exposure in the womb, and to early childhood conditioning.

The qualities that need to be checked when examining the digits are their stiffness, lower phalange size, and knottiness, and a comparison of the length of the index and ring fingers.

Finger flexibility

Finger flexibility is a reflection of mental flexibility. Simply put, rigid digits are indicative of a rigid mind and hyperflexive ones show a butterfly mind.

Stiffness of the fingers is checked by simply wrapping your own fingers around the fingers of the person you're reading for, and, while holding their wrist with your other hand, gently pushing all the digits back towards the wrist until resistance is felt (Figure 6.1).

The average flexibility is for all the digits to move back together from the vertical by around 5 cm. If that is the case, it's normal and of no consequence.

Fingers that don't move back at all when you push against them show high internal stress, rigid mental processes, and a lack of

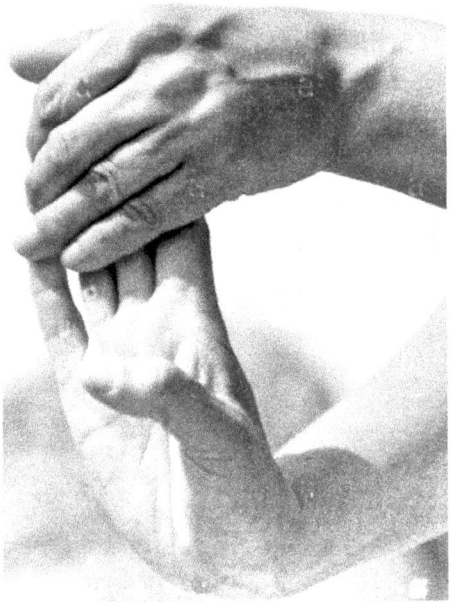

Figure 6.1. Testing the fingers' flexibility.

spontaneity. This can be positive in an area of life where conformity, fixed patterns, and regimented procedures are useful, like the military. However, this is one of the primary stress indicators, and other signs of stress in the palm can be sought to confirm this. Often rigid fingers are a sign that a person finds it difficult to relax and is somewhat locked up internally, which can lead to many disorders if not dealt with. They need to release stress physically by, for example, yoga and deep tissue massage. If the digits are painful to move backwards and if accompanied by swelling of the knuckles of the lowest finger joints, this is an early classic indication of rheumatoid arthritis in its first stages, particularly if the lower joints become red and warm. Contrastingly, osteoarthritis, or the mild, "wear and tear" form of the disease, tends to involve swelling of the joints nearest the tops of the fingers, with pain when pulled back and but no redness or heat.

Floppy digits

Where the fingers are floppy and bend back 45° or more, it shows an impulsive mind. Open, spontaneous, and expressive, this is a person receptive to new ideas but psychologically all over the place, never sticking to any view, value, or opinion for long. Flexible digits are perfectly normal on children's hands and common on the hands of free-thinking artists, dancers, and dilettantes. Though very loose finger movement usually indicates a flexible and mobile spine, hips, and shoulders, this has been linked to long-term joint issues, and particularly to spinal disc problems, hip joint over-extension damage, and general joint problems from middle age onward. The key with hyper flexible fingers (and very flexible body joints) is to develop strategies to strengthen the muscle and connective tissue around the major articulation points of the body through such practices as yoga and Pilates. The emphasis should always be on building strength rather than extending joints further.

The finger phalanges

The three sections of the fingers separated by joint creases are known as phalanges. Of particular interest in health analysis are the lower finger phalanges.

If the base phalanges are all disproportionately large (Figure 6.2), the sensual, physical, and material realms are naturally exaggerated in that person's life. To put it quite simply, those with overly large base phalanges have enormous drives to satiate their love of sensual pleasure (including sexual gratification). They get great joy from feeling, tasting, and touching. Those with over-large base phalanges tend to have great battles with their weight, and here can be seen the link between sexual gratification and physical pleasure (or the lack of it) and weight gain.

This can be a particular issue if the hand is an earth shape (giving a naturally broad body type that is never meant to be thin), and if the thumb is floppy and the Venus mount flat. This presents a lifelong struggle to keep weight in check against the vast panoply of temptations of the commercial food industry. Where you find this sort of issue on a pair of hands, it's vital that any

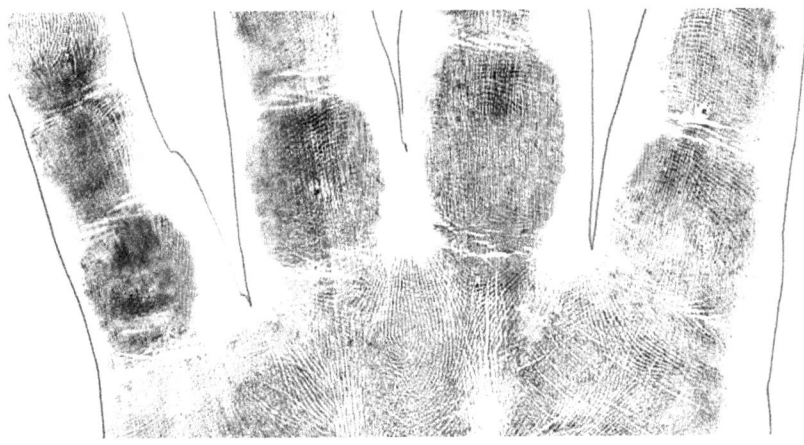

Figure 6.2. Large basal phalanges.

diet programme is one that allows tasty treats and is compensated with sensual experiences like beauty treatments, pampering, and massage. Sexual issues should be explored. Only via a pleasurable route can healthy goals be attained.

Relative ring and index finger length

The next point to examine is the difference in length between the index and the third (ring) finger. This is known as the 2D:4D (2nd digit versus 4th digit) ratio and is one of the most intensely studied aspects of the hands in medical and scientific studies. In palmistry, the index finger is by far the most important, as it is the finger representing the ego, identity, sense of self, self-esteem, and self-value. On the passive hand, it is a powerful reflector of the relationship a person has had with the primary carer figure in their upbringing, and its size relative to the ring finger is crucial.

The ring finger is about the persona, performance, the public face, and the need for attention. It is believed to be part of our personality that seeks to flirt, to display and demonstrate an edge in the primal drive to acquire a high-status mate. Many studies have shown that the length of these two digits is a crucial indicator of testosterone (ring) and oestrogen (index) exposure in the womb and to the influence of the primary parental figure in infancy.

In general, females tend to have longer index fingers than males, though this will vary enormously between individuals. Almost all studies discovered developmental and medical issues if the ring finger is significantly (by 2 cm or more) longer than the index finger (Figure 6.3). It must always be borne in mind that when the ring finger is long, the index is always consequently short. This means that the sense of self-esteem and self-value is eclipsed by the persona and performance aspect of the personality.

The ring finger being over 2 cm longer than the index has been linked to better performance in sports, the need for media and public attention, musical ability, risk-taking, injury through car

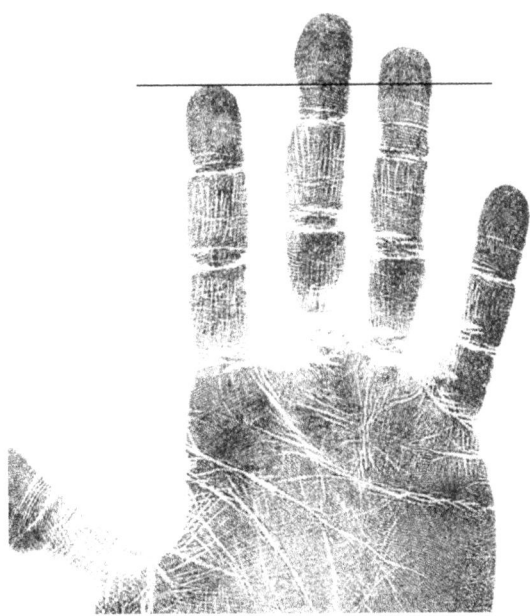

Figure 6.3. Long ring digit.

accidents and dangerous sports, heart disease, amphetamine and cocaine dependence, and smoking-induced lung cancer. In males it increases the risk of prostate cancer and male-pattern baldness. In two studies, the long ring showed a four times higher than average rate of hair loss by age 40. This digit being long is also linked to a higher risk of being unfaithful to one's partner. (Hashemian et al., "2D:4D-Ratios among Individuals …"; Kasielska-Trojan et al., "Digit Ratios and Their Asymmetries …")

In females, the long ring finger has been indicated in high-performance sports and in outstanding creative and musical expression, as well as in anxiety and depression, knee and hip osteoarthritis, breast cancer, obesity, addiction, and, again, less likely to be faithful to a partner. (Finley et al., "Born to be wild")

There are three important points to be borne in mind here. First, testosterone levels in females are on average 15 times lower than in males, so the effect of the long ring digit on females is weaker and more internalised. Second, the low self-esteem and poor self-value indicated by the short index digit may well be at the root of many of the health issues, so counselling and raising self-belief may well moderate the health picture enormously. Lastly, the disease risk issues raised here are statistically significant, but the fact is that the majority of people with a long ring finger will not get the health problems indicated in the research.

Trigger finger

Approximately 3% of the population develop trigger finger. This is more common in women and most often occurs after the age of 50. Its proper name is stenosing tenosynovitis. It occurs when a tendon becomes too inflamed to easily slide through the hand's joints. When the condition is advanced, a swollen, tender lump appears on the inner palm side. It is far more common on the ring finger or thumb than on the other digits. It is more likely in those who have diabetes, thyroid issues, or rheumatoid arthritis, so it's worth investigating other indications of these problems on other parts of the hands.

Sources

Finley, B., Kalwij, A., & Kapteyn, A. "Born to be wild: Second-to-fourth digit length ratio and risk preferences." *Economics and Human Biology,* Vol. 47 (2022): 101178.

Hashemian, S. S., Golshani, S., et al. "2D:4D-ratios among individuals with amphetamine use disorder, antisocial personality disorder and with both amphetamine use disorder and antisocial personality disorder." *Journal of Psychiatric Research,* Vol. 170 (2024): 81–89.

Kasielska-Trojan, A., Manning, J. T., et al., "Digit ratios and their asymmetries as risk factors of developmental instability and hospitalization." *Scientific Reports,* Vol. 12, No. 4573 (2022).

7

Fingerprint patterns

An enormous amount of research has taken place on finger and palm print patterns. Some 12,000 papers have been published on particular print formations on the palm and fingers being linked to dispositions towards diseases. Epidermal ridges (the raised skin lines that form prints) are formed between 11 and 24 weeks of gestation; after this period the ridges do not change, except for slight fading in very old age as the skin becomes thinner and less pronounced. The scientific term for the print patterns are dermatoglyphics (from the Greek, derma: skin; glyphics: markings). Although the term "dermatoglyphics" was coined by Cummins and Midlo in their breakthrough book, *Fingerprints, Palms and Soles*, in 1961, dermatoglyphics as a scientific discipline began with the publication of Francis Galton's classic work, *Finger Prints*, in 1892. Even though the primary object of Galton's studies was to develop a personal identification system, he investigated the biological variation of fingerprints and the unchangeable characteristics of the patterns through time. It was from Galton's research that the United Kingdom developed the fingerprint classifications still used today in criminal investigations. Interest in dermatoglyphic research continued unabated from the beginning of the twentieth century, but dermatoglyphics entered into a phase of rapid expansion from the 1960s onward, attracting a great number of scientists from all segments of biology, medicine, and biological anthropology.

Fingerprints are massively important in modern palmistry. Though they are practically unknown in any palmistry book written before 1970, they are so vital in reading character that some schools of palmistry focus only on fingerprints and ignore everything else!

The five print patterns

Let us start with an exploration of the types of print patterns and their meanings psychologically. The metaphor palmists use to visualise the print patterns is as brain waves, representing currents of thought. Fingerprints allow hand readers to know the manner of a person's thinking. We cannot know what they are thinking, but the prints give us an understanding of the way someone processes information.

Every print on every palm is an original and unique marking, but all print patterns fall into five broad types.

These five print patterns are the whorl, simple arch, tented arch, loop, and double loop composite.

Whorl prints: the vortex

The whorl (Figure 7.1) is made of a series of ever-decreasing circles or a spiral that curls into itself. Whorls concentrate and fix the flow of mental energy in a central torrent of thought, hence its vortex metaphor. Sometimes there are a few loop lines wrapped around the whorl, which can make it more difficult to identify. The whorl shows mental patterns that spin in a highly targeted manner, rather like the rings around a bullseye. Whorl patterns are more common on males.

A whorl makes for an intensely focused and often an obsessive mindset and gives a need for space, privacy, and the drive to be alone and unsupervised. Whorls are highly secretive, freedom-

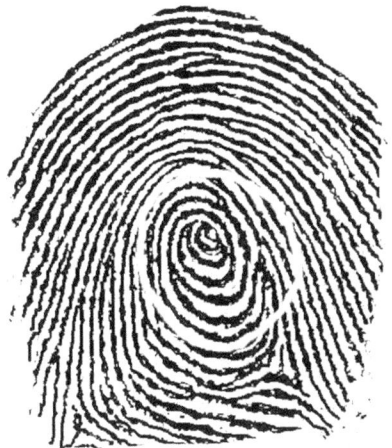

Figure 7.1. Whorl print.

loving, odd, and eccentric. Where there are whorls on many fingers, they make for an inventive and highly original personality who is uninterested in following trends, fashions, and groups.

The whorl is seen in abundance on talented people. It isn't, on its own, a sign of creativity, but it signals originality, an analytical mind, a lack of a herd instinct, and the ability to be alone for long periods, which is the basis for any creative expression. Whorls are rarely found on group performers, like actors, who must obey script or director; they are much more likely on the writer or the screenwriter.

The nature of the whorl means that deep focus on one particular subject is far preferable to a broad set of skills, so this makes for a nature that has a specialist interest or hobby; multi-whorled people usually become experts or specialists. Whorls give an ability to avoid group-think, and whorl-dominant types often are often perceived as being loners or antisocial.

Whenever you see a lot of whorls on a palm, it's inevitable that that person will spend the majority of their lives alone – even if married with four children, they will find a way to isolate themselves for long periods of time.

Simple arch print: ocean floor

The simple arch is a flat chevron shape, made of a series of inverted "V" lines piled on top of each other (Figure 7.2). The thought patterns are linear, simple, and direct, built on practical, well-proven, traditional lines. The simple arch tends to thought patterns that resonate to the past, the known, the fixed and pragmatic, and is related to the drive to seek solidity and connect to base. Simple arches are more common on females.

People with simple arches don't like abstract, fanciful ideas: their mindset is realistic and based on the physical realm. The simple arch is a sign of a repressive personality – someone fixed, faithful, deep, loyal, dependable, and practical. In terms of employment, the person with many simple arches is going to have far fewer days off, will be more reliable, and will stick to jobs far longer than people with other print patterns. Their work will tend to be secure, routine-orientated, with a pension, rather than something high-risk.

Simple arches indicate an obsession with the home and family and with financial security. Their need to repress emotion can mean it's hard for them to show vulnerability or to let off steam,

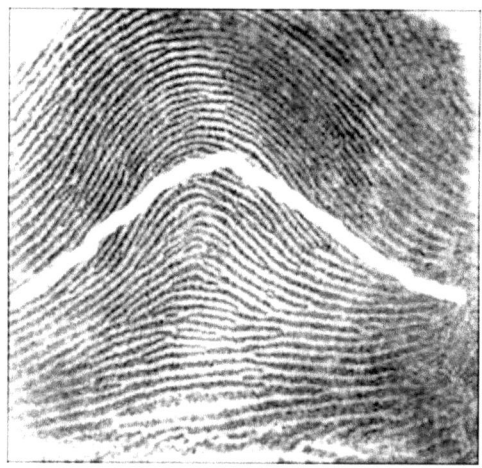

Figure 7.2. A simple arch.

and they need to express their inner tensions through physical activity. They can get stuck in worn-out routines and can often hold themselves back, hesitant to grab opportunities.

The simple arch indicates the impulse to protect, defend, and save animals, nature, vulnerable people, and the oppressed. It is common on those who serve the community in some way and those whose work is concerned with children, family, animals, or preserving the environment.

Someone with a simple arch is highly tribal, so there is enormous loyalty to one's group, tribe, family, substitute family, or friends.

This pattern lends the ability to use one's hands, so it's common on craftspeople and those who shape, mould, and repair. Simple-arch-dominant people are obsessed with their home and are great house doer-uppers and home decorators.

The simple arch person will put family and financial security before everything. Such a person is incapable of being snobby or pretentious and, however wealthy, will always possess a common touch.

The simple arch has an issue psychologically about fairness and equality and is very anti anything where there is an elite, monopoly, privileged class, or ruling clique.

Tented arch print: the tidal wave

Tented arches are the rarest print pattern, but are easily recognised by the distinctive "spike" formation in the centre, like a tent pole with the other lines "pushed" up around it (Figure 7.3). Sometimes there is a slim loop pattern alongside the spike, but if the sharp upward stroke is in the centre of the fingertip, seeming to push the loop to the side, it's a tented arch. Conceptually, the tented arch is high-minded, intense, and passionate, with great peaks of focus that quickly die away.

Tented arches are indicators of an intense personality. Just one of these markers on a hand indicates an excitable mindset that leaps high in dramatic directions. A tented arch is opportunistic

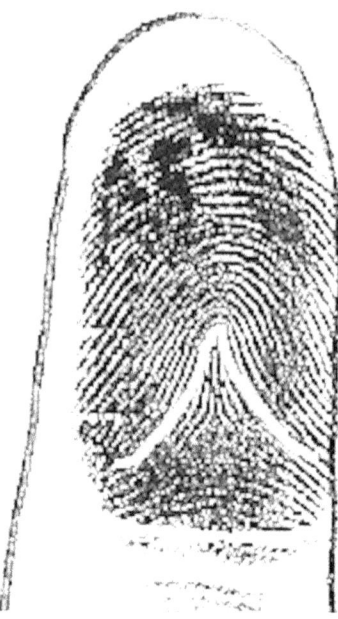

Figure 7.3. Tented arch print.

and gives a drive to be exceptional in some way. Psychologically, this pattern shows a need to lift oneself into a higher, more elevated realm.

Those with a tented arch need to stand out and above other people, either by being inspiring teachers, innovators, leaders, rebels, performers, or motivators, or by guiding others to more adventurous realms.

There is a strong drive to lift, dramatise, shock, and excite. Tented arch people are never boring: they have a need to push themselves beyond normal boundaries and to transform themselves, so they are highly adventurous, quick-thinking, and responsive.

Those with this pattern need both an exciting outlet for their energies and a need to learn how to relax.

The ulnar loop: tidal flow

By far the most common pattern you'll come across on the fingertips is the ulnar loop. Ulnar loops are thrown in the direction of the thumb; they rise and fall like waves (Figure 7.4). Over 70% of all the prints you'll see on hands will be ulnar loops. The loop is about going with the flow, responding to others, with empathy to one's group, family, and environment. Loopy people tend to be highly responsive to others and to be in tune with current trends, fashions, and beliefs, hence the tide metaphor. Those in group arts, such as band members, actors, dancers, and so on, always have an abundance of loops, as do people-people, carers, and highly sociable souls. Generally, loops are seen as the most contented of

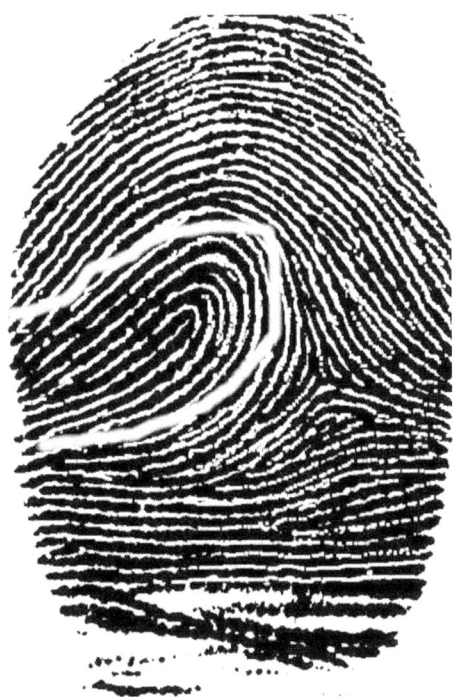

Figure 7.4. Print of a right-hand index-finger ulnar loop: the flow of the loop is towards the thumb.

patterns, as it's about fitting in and prioritising friendships and relationships. Don't assume that loopy people are boring and ultra-"normal". They may well be involved in the arts, or be part of a rock band, or a professional surfing champion. It is just that the flow of the ulnar loop means the brain functions extremely well in responding to the flow, zeitgeist, trend, sense, and rhythm of their environment.

Radial loops: raging rip tide

Radial loops are highly significant and are much rarer than ulnar loops. In shape and form they are exactly the same as ulnar loops, except that they move in the opposite direction, flowing away from the thumb (Figure 7.5). It is easy to see the difference, as the radial loop flows towards the little finger and points away from the thumb on either hand. For this reason it is often called the "reversed loop" or "wrong-way-round loop".

The radial loop creates hyper-responsiveness to other people, and an enormous drive to be liked and be accepted. There's always an over-sensitivity to being criticised or being at fault. It is

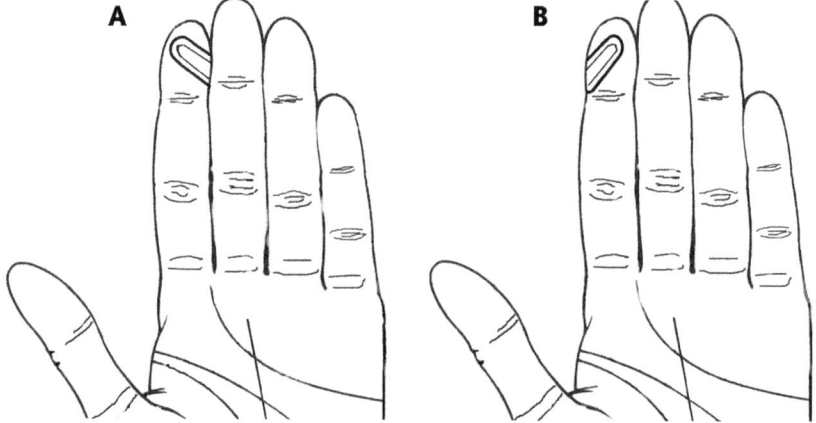

Figure 7.5. (A) Ulnar loop. (B) Radial loop. The ulnar loop flows towards the thumb; the radial loop flows away from the thumb.

as if the loop in this reverse direction makes one get caught in the tide of other's energy, and this interferes with the person's psychological stability.

This pattern is often found on the pleaser, flatterer, or enabler. These are often called "carer's loops as ideal vocation for the radial loop is some kind of therapist, advisor, medical professional or HR manager. The radial pattern is a sign of a need to avoid negativity from other people and develop a great capacity to get in tune with anyone. There's an innately insecure, hyper-receptive sense of identity. This is a very important sign and needs to be understood by the bearer. It can be a source of difficulty on any hand, but it's particularly destabilising on a bendy-thumbed water hand. The loop turned outwards absorbs everything from outside; such people are in danger of defining themselves only in response to other people. Criticism can be devastating for bearers of this sign, but when given the support and praise they crave, they can achieve much.

Being so receptive means the radial looped person can "tune in" intuitively to others. On a thick-skinned fire hand, this can indicate an aggressive, highly defensive person who feels constantly "under attack" and who can be prone to paranoia and antisocial behaviour. These people internalise others' needs as their own and can be guilty of being what others want, rather than what they themselves are. Advice should always be given to spend more time alone and develop self-knowledge. Radial loop people often seek constant life changes, as they have a chameleon-like quality that changes to suit different environments.

Composite prints: two tides

The composite is formed by two loops going in opposite directions, like the yin-yang symbol of the Tao (Figure 7.6). This is considered a spiritual sign in Eastern cultures. The two loops form two waves in opposition to each other, and so this pattern is a sign of psychological dualism, doubt, uncertainty, and never being able to

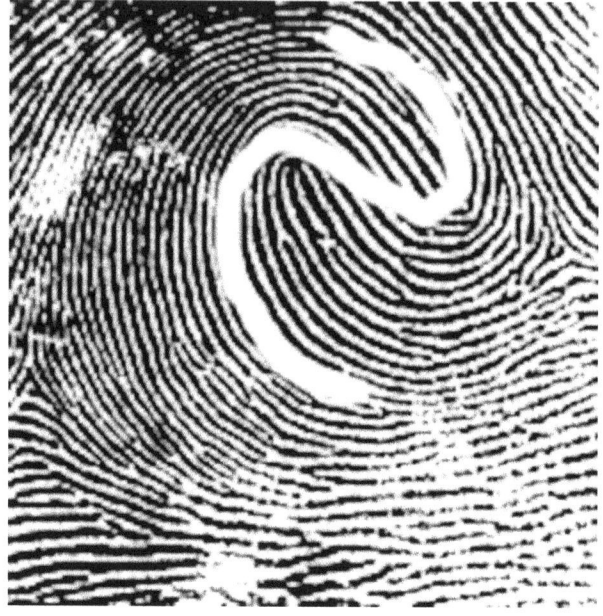

Figure 7.6. Composite.

fully commit. The mental patterns flow in two different directions, rather than as a direct current to a clear conclusion.

This is a distinctly helpful sign on anyone who is in a position of looking at all sides of any issue and being non-judgemental – for example a counsellor, legal representative, judge, academic, or advisor.

Where this sign is found, there is always a fascination with philosophy and spiritual practice and a natural drive to be non-judgemental. This sign means that a person cannot be hurried to a conclusion and will always be ambivalent: it can be highly frustrating on a fire palm to have such doubt, which often manifests as someone jumping from one ambition to another, but when placed in a situation where multiple viewpoints are needed, it's a powerful gift.

Deciphering the dermatoglyphics

It will help you enormously to memorise and understand the print patterns by visualising them as waves of thought. The pattern of the print replicates the thinking process.

Understand the simple arch as indicating thinking in simple, pragmatic lines, not jumping to conclusions. Ideas are built on the foundation of the simple, demonstrable, natural, tried, and trusted.

Those with tented arches make fantastic leaps upward into the possible, potential, ideal, and inspirational.

Whorls twist ideas around and around in a deeply focused way, always having their own angle on anything.

Composites balance opposing waves of thought: they see two sides to any idea.

Radial loops are like wind socks that are blown around by exterior stimuli: they are hyper-responsive to other people, peer pressure, and their environment.

Sources

Cummins, H., & Midlo, C. *Fingerprints, Palms and Soles: An Introduction to Dermatoglyphics* (New York: Dover, 1943, 1961).
Galton. F. *Finger Prints* (London: MacMillan, 1892).

8

Dermatoglyphics and disease

Since the 1970s, there has been extensive study into linking particular fingerprint patterns as predictors of the likelihood of disease and as an "early-warning" system to make intervention more successful.

The vast library of studies and reports can sometimes be contradictory and can vary across gender, age, and racial types. Some studies are simply too small to be of worth. Only where there is a substantial link from print patterns to illness across many investigations are they reported here. It is fascinating to see how the psychological profile of a print pattern so often gives rise to an equivalent issue in the body. As always, manifesting with a particular set of print patterns indicates only a statistically higher likelihood of a disease. The majority of people with a given pattern will *not* develop the disease. In 1976, Blanka Schaumann and Milton Alter published *Dermatoglyphics in Medical Disorders*, an excellent summary of the findings of dermatoglyphic patterns and subsequent disease.

Fingerprint patterns

Simple arch

A high number of simple arches (4 or more) indicates a higher incidence of foetal developmental issues: Patau's syndrome and Edwards syndrome. There is also a higher risk of chronic gastrointestinal obstruction, constipation, rheumatoid arthritis, and cervical cancer.

Whorl

A large number of whorl prints (more than five) is associated with a higher risk of Turner's syndrome, bronchial asthma, myopia, over-sensitivity to light, and heart disease through hypertension. One study found that for every whorl print, systolic blood pressure increased by 2.2 mmHg, so this is clearly an issue where multi-whorled people need to take steps to keep blood pressure in check. Obsessive behaviour, paranoia, and schizophrenia were also indicated.

A high number of whorls on females' hands indicated a higher incidence of breast cancer.

Loops

A number of studies have indicated that nine or ten loops indicate a higher risk of Alzheimer's disease and late-onset dementia, as well as rheumatoid arthritis and immune-system disorders.

Radial loops

If radial loops are present, they are likely to be on the index digit. There is evidence of increased incidence of depression and paranoia in males and body issues, like bulimia and anorexia, on females. Rapidly progressive periodontis (RPP) was also indicated in both genders.

Composite

There is no definitive medical issue with a composite print except for the very rare incidence of a composite occurring on the palm – not on a finger or the thumb (Figure 8.1). This very occasionally is seen in the lower hand quadrant, opposite the Venus mount. This was shown to be prevalent in a higher incidence of Turner's syndrome and Klinefelter syndrome, conditions that affect sexual development: Turner's syndrome if the person is a female who has masculine features, and Klinefelter syndrome in a male who has some feminine characteristics. Usually these conditions cannot be recognised until after puberty, once the sexual characteristics are fully developed.

Though not reported in scientific journals, many palm readers have made a connection between a composite print on the palm and development of schizophrenia.

Tented arch

Tented arches are the rarest prints and, if found, will usually be present on the index digit. This is associated with mania, obsessive behaviour, heart palpitations, and heart arrhythmia.

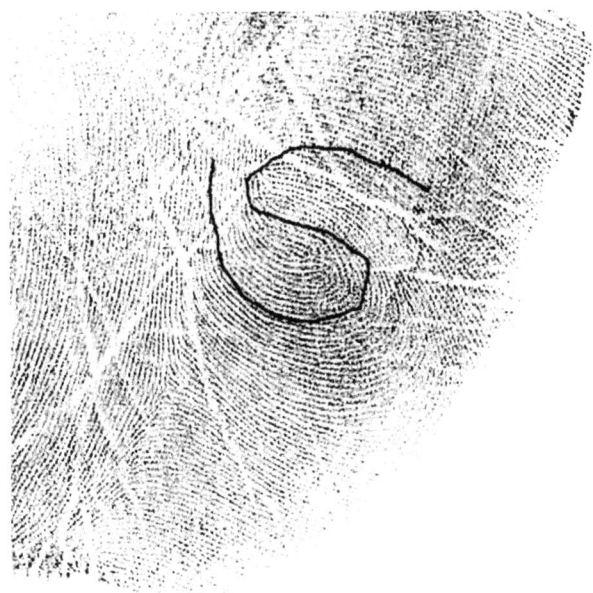

Figure 8.1. Composite print on the palm.

Triradius

An important marking of interest in print patterns and disease is the axial triradius: a meeting point of skin ridges that resembles a three-way junction at the base of the palm. The triradius is usually observed at the base near the wrist. However, on the hands of people with an "autosomal trisomy" (associated with congenital malformations that may result in prolonged hospitalisation of the new-born), the axial triradius is found at a higher region of the palm.

The raised triradius (Figure 8.2) is also a significant pointer to congenital heart disease. Various studies have noted that the frequency of higher placement of the palmar axial triradii in either hand occurred with significantly greater frequency in patients with congenital heart disease (most studies found the figure to be

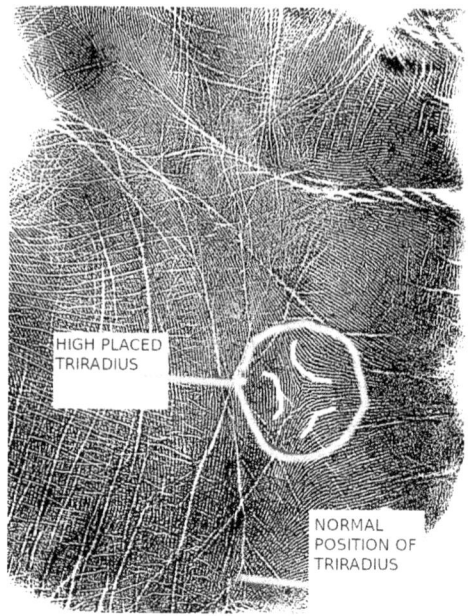

Figure 8.2. Normal and raised axial triradius.

60–70% of patients with this marker). Large studies in India and among Japanese–Hawaiians found that almost three quarters of male patients with congenital heart disease had a displaced triradius that was halfway up the palm in comparison to less than 20% in the control group.

Sources

Schaumann, B., & Alter, M. *Dermatoglyphics in Medical Disorders* (New York: Springer Verlag, 1976), pp. 187–189.

Simple arch
Babler, W. J. "Embryological development of epidermal ridges and their configuration." *Birth Defects Original Article Series*, Vol. 27, No. 2 (1991): 95–112
Bonnevie, K. "Studies on papillary pattern of human fingers." *Journal of Genetics*, Vol. 15 (1924): 1–11.
Chakraborty, R. "The role of heredity and environment on dermatoglyphic traits." *Birth Defects Original Article Series*, Vol. 27, No. 2 (1991): 151–191.

Floris, G., Sanciu, M. G., & Sanna, E. "Dermatoglyphics in pathology with emphasis on breast cancer and cervix carcinoma: Some results." *International Journal of Anthropology*, Vol. 5, No. 2 (1990), pp. 125–128.

Plato, C. C., Garruto, R. M., & Schaumann, B. A. (Eds.), *Dermatoglyphics: Science in Transition* (New York: Wiley-Liss, 1991).

Pulliam, T. J., & Schuster, M. M. "Congenital markers for chronic intestinal obstruction." *American Journal of Gastroenterology*, Vol. 90 (1995): 922–926.

Ravindranath, R., Shubha, R., Nagesh, H. V., Johnson, J., & Rajangam, S. "Dermatoglyphics in rheumatoid arthritis." *Indian Journal of Medical Sciences*, Vol. 57, No. 10 (2003): 437–441.

Whorl

Godfrey, K. M., Barker, D. J., Peace, J., Cloke, J., & Osmond, C. "Relation of fingerprints and shape of the palm to fetal growth and adult blood pressure." *British Medical Journal*, Vol. 307 (1993): 405–408.

Gupta, U. K., & Prakash, S. "Dermatoglyphics: A study of finger tip patterns in bronchial asthma and its genetic disposition." *Kathmandu University Medical Journal*, Vol. 1, No. 4 (2003): 267–271.

Lubovitz, O. S., Trattner, A., Katznelson, M. B. M., & Sandbank, M. "Dermatoglyphics in Darters disease". *International Journal of Dermatology*, Vol. 33, No. 9 (2007): 626–627.

Mulvihill, J. J., & Smith, D. W. "The genesis of dermatoglyphics." *Journal of Pediatrics*, Vol. 75 (1969): 579–589.

Oladipo, G. S., Olotu, E. J., Fawehinmi, H. B., Okoh, P. D., & Iboroma, A. D. "Dermatoglyphics in idiopathic (primary) dilated cardiomyopathy in Southern Nigeria." *Scientific Research and Essays*, Vol. 2, No. 10 (2007): 416-420.

Loops

Cummins, H., & Midlo, C. *Fingerprints, Palms and Soles: An Introduction to Dermatoglyphics* (New York: Dover, 1943, 1961).

Cummins, H., & Midlo, C. "Palmar and planter epidermal configuration (dermatoglyphics) in European-Americans." *American Journal of Physical Anthropology*, Vol. 9 (1926): 471–502.

Harrison, G. A. *Genetical Variations in Human Populations* (Oxford: Pergamon, 1961). PP791.

Pulliam, T. J., & Schuster, M. M. "Congenital markers for chronic intestinal obstruction." *American Journal of Gastroenterology*, Vol. 90 (1995): 922–926.

Rajangam, S., Ravindranth, R., Shubha, R., Nagesh, H. V., & Johnson, J. (2008). Dermatoglyphics-Quantitative Analysis in Rheumatoid Arthritis. *The Anthropologist*, 10(3), 233–235

Singh, P. K., Pandey, S. S., & Singh, G. (1987). "Dermatoglyphics in auto-immune dermatoses." *Indian Journal of Dermatology*, Vol. 32 , No. 1 (1987): 15–18.

Terry, R. D., & Katzman, R. "Senile dementia of the Alzheimer type." *Annals of Neurology*, Vol. 14, No. 5 (1983): 497–506.

Walker, J. F. A. "Sex linked recessive finger print pattern." *Journal of Heredity*, Vol. 32 (1964): 279–280.

Radial loops

Achs, R., Harper, R. G., & Siegel, M. "Unusual dermatophytic findings associated with rubella embryopathy." *New England Journal of Medicine*, Vol. 274 (1966): 148–150.

Atasu, M., Kuru, B., Firatli, E., et al. "Dermatoglyphic findings in periodontal diseases." *International Journal of Anthropology*, Vol. 20, Nos. 1–2 (2005): 6375.

Cambell, E. *Fingerprints and Behaviour: A Text on Fingerprints and Behavioural Correspondences, Volume 1* (Seattle, WA: Amida Biometrics, 1998).

Composite
Cambell, E. *Fingerprints and Behaviour: A Text on Fingerprints and Behavioural Correspondences, Volume 1* (Seattle, WA: Amida Biometrics, 1998).

Tented arch
Cambell, E. *Fingerprints and Behaviour: A Text on Fingerprints and Behavioural Correspondences, Volume 1* (Seattle, WA: Amida Biometrics, 1998).
Holt, S. B. *The Genetics of Dermal Ridges* (Springfield, IL: Charles C Thomas, 1968).
Lacroix, B., Wolff-Quenot, M. J., & Haffen, K. (1984). "Early human hand morphology: an estimation of fetal age." *Early Human Development*, Vol. 9, No. 2 (1984): 127–136
Sontakke, B. R., Ghosh, S. K., & Pal, A. K. "Dermatoglyphics of fingers and palm in Klinefelter's syndrome." *Nepal Medical College Journal*, Vol. 12, No.3 (2010):142–144.

Triradius
Cummins, H., & Midlo, C. *Fingerprints, Palms and Soles: An Introduction to Dermatoglyphics* (New York: Dover, 1943, 1961).
Cummins, H., Talley, C., & Platou. R. V. "Palmar dermatoglyphics in mongolism." *Pediatrics*, Vol. 5, No. 2: 241–248.
Floris, G. "Dermatoglyphics in cases of hypospadias: New data." *International Journal of Anthropology*, Vol. 8 (1993): 39–41.
Floris, G., Sanciu, M. G., & Sanna, E. "Dermatoglyphics in pathology with emphasis on breast cancer and cervix carcinoma: Some results." *International Journal of Anthropology*, Vol. 5, No. 2 (1990), pp. 125–128.
JAMA. "The hand and cardiovascular disease." *Journal of the American Medical Association*, Vol. 154, No. 6 (1994): 508.
Lacroix, B., Wolff-Quenot, M. J., & Haffen, K. (1984). Early human hand morphology: An estimation of fetal age. *Early Human Development*, Vol. 9: 127–136.
Lu, H., Qian, W., Geng, Z., Sheng, Y., Yu, H., et al. "Dermatoglyphs in coronary artery disease among Ningxia population of North China." *Journal of Clinical and Diagnostic Research*, Vol. 9, No. 12 (2015): AC01–4.
Plato, C. C., Garruto, R. M., & Schaumann, B. A. (Eds.). *Dermatoglyphics: Science in Transition (Second Edition)*, (New York: Wiley-Liss), 1991).
Shamai-Lubovitz, O., Trattner, A., Katznelson, M. B., & Sandbank, M. "Dermatoglyphics in Darier's disease." *International Journal of Dermatology*, Vol. 33, No. 9 (1994): 626–627.
Takashina, T., & Yorifuji, S. "Palmar dermatoglyphics in heart disease. Differential studies in Japanese and American populations with congenital and acquired heart diseases." *Journal of the American Medical Association*, Vol. 197, No. 9 (1966): 689–692.

9

The major lines

We now move on to the palm lines. These lines are crucial in health analysis, as they are representative of different energy pathways. The lines show the attitudes, priorities, and values that drive us and that eventually lead to physical manifestations. Rather like a wiring diagram of a house, the palm's major lines indicate which circuits are operating well, poorly, or barely at all. It is relatively easy to spot signs of problems years in advance of stethoscope or blood test. Like wiring, the body takes time to fail, and usually in the case of major lines signs appear decades before issues arise. And, because lines change, taking preventive action will head off a condition before it becomes manifest. The palm's lines can show us exactly in what area of life and in what parts of the body an issue is brewing, and with the right diet, exercise, rest, and therapy, the line's quality and the problem can be remedied.

There is little in the way of serious medical studies on the health implications of lines of the palm, as the scientific community is wary of the superstition that still lingers over the idea that lines predict events. Most evidence is supplied by my own and other hand readers' experience, by medically qualified hand readers like Eugene Schienmann, and investigative hand readers like Nathaniel Altman and Noel Jaquin.

There are four major lines that are present in some rudimentary form on the palms of almost all adults. Each of the main lines has an elementary quality – earth, water, fire, and air (traditionally named life, heart, head, and fate) lines. Each relates to a different area of human experience.

First of all, let's take a look at the four major lines.

The major lines vary enormously in length, quality and strength, and any hand you examine, including your own, will have lines that look very different from the image below – they may be shorter, fainter, or more splintered in form but will be roughly in the same position as those in Figure 9.1.

The lines form between the ninth and eleventh weeks of gestation and change slowly throughout one's lifetime. Many palmists read for the same person every couple of years, as their lineal patterns change.

Figure 9.2 shows typical line changes over a period of five years.

If the hand shape, skin texture, and fingerprints form the fixed, genetic, unchanging aspect of human beings, the lines are the mutable responses to life experience.

In addition to the major lines, there are nearly always other minor lines present.

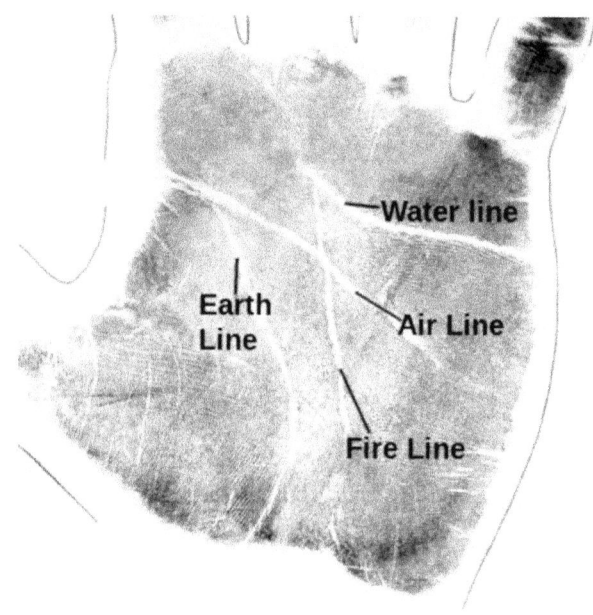

Figure 9.1. The major lines.

THE MAJOR LINES

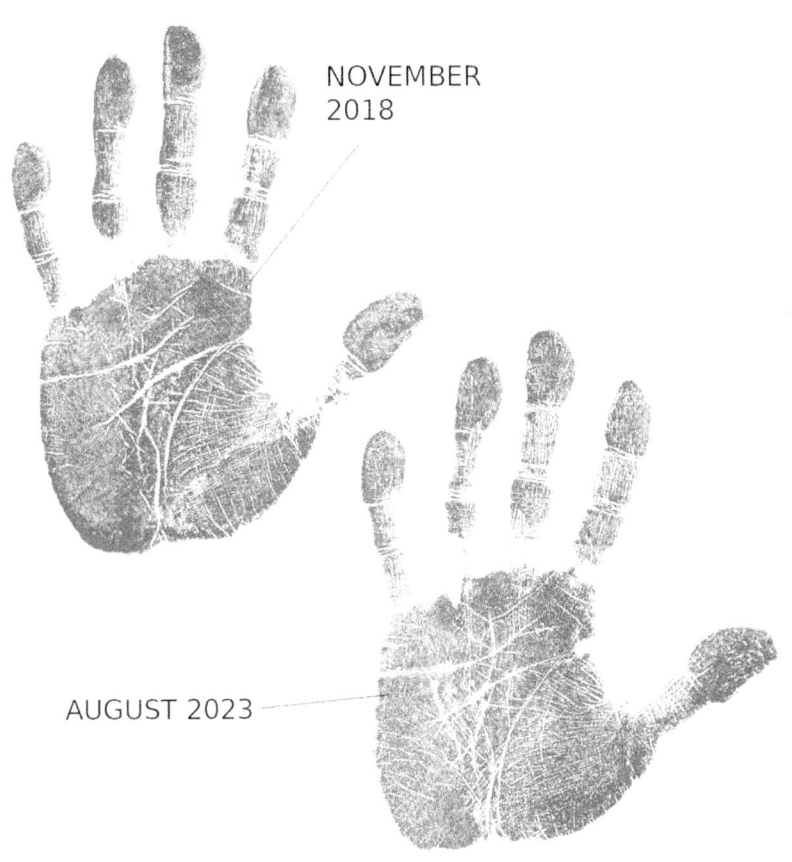

Figure 9.2. Line changes.

Basic principles of the lines

The flow of any line should ideally be like that of a free-flowing river, unimpeded by islands, bar lines, or breaks. In this respect, a very thick, trench-like line is similar to a silted-up river, and a faint, broken up line is like a trickle that has poor flow. In either case, the function of the line will be poor and the energetic potential limited.

It is quite normal to have at least one major line that is of somewhat poor quality – we humans aren't perfect in every level of life – almost always there is a realm in which we are vulnerable. Even if a major line is in very poor condition, the person can function perfectly well, as other lines (and areas of strength) will compensate to some extent. A poor, broken-up, or very weak major line may indicate less-than-absolute optimum health, but likely not an illness or health problem until at least middle age or later. It is very important to emphasise this point, as the old idea of lines predicting ghastly outcomes is still a hard one to shake off. A poor-quality line will take a very long time before it becomes a chronic health problem. Lines are much more indicative of the attitudes, behaviour, and drives that create a medical issue. Our mindset and behaviour is where we can work to remedy an issue. You might see a line as a sort of flow of healing energy. If the line is weak and broken, the protective power is poor, and one is more vulnerable in that area.

Super-strong, deep, red lines can also present a difficulty in that they are overworking and overloading in some way. A major line often stands out as being much stronger than the others, and this shows an over-emphasis on a particular area of experience and a certain organic overload. If, for instance, the water line (which relates to emotional flow) is very strong and deep and red while all the other lines are fainter, this means that physical energy and stability (earth line), goals and direction (fire line), and mental clarity (air line) are all at the mercy of how the person is feeling. This would have a bearing on health, as the person could easily develop an illness or psychological condition if, for instance, a crisis emerges in personal relationships.

All the lines in our hands are in our power to change. New patterns of behaviour and, particularly, complementary therapies and an openness to adapt new ways of being will head off most physical issues.

The long and the short: the length of lines

Major lines can be too long or too short. A short line (extending less than halfway across the palm) means there is a short, limited energy in a particular realm, and that line's power and reach is limited in scope. A major line can also be too long. If it crosses the palm from side to side or top to bottom to completely bisect the palm at any point, this creates a compulsion of some sort. It cuts the hand in half and creates an obsessive short-circuit to over-think (air line), over-feel (water line), overwork (fire line) or over extend the body (earth line).

Beginnings and endings

All the major lines start at the same point on the palm but vary hugely in where they end (Figure 9.3). The earth line begins above the thumb on the side of the palm and runs in a semicircle downwards. The water line begins under the little finger and runs horizontally towards the index digit. The fire line begins in the bottom half of the palm and runs through the centre of the palm up towards the middle finger. The air line begins very close to or at the same point as the earth line and runs horizontally across the middle of the palm.

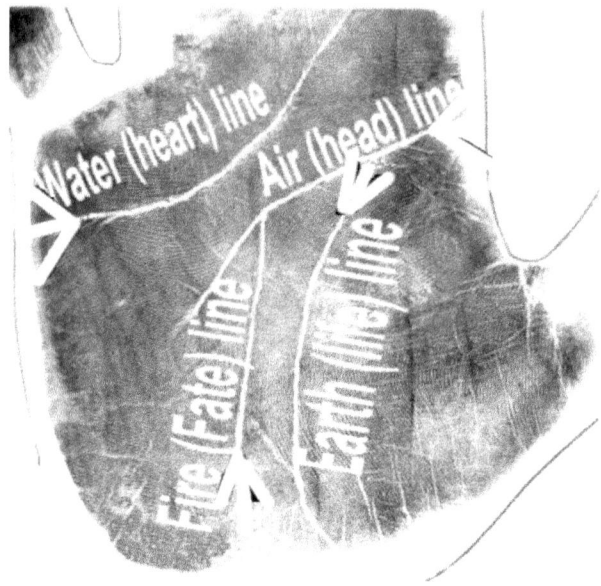

Figure 9.3. Major line beginning points.

10

The major earth line

The meaning, metaphor, and nature of the earth line

The earth line marks the foundations of a person's being and is always the first line to examine in health terms. It was traditionally called the lifeline, as it was assumed that the length of the line foretold the length of a person's life. Having studied the lines of many elderly people, I can assure you that there are thousands in their eighties with short earth lines alive and well, complaining about their chilblains!

The way to think of this line is as a root, starting above the thumb, curving around the thumb ball, embedding itself into the base at the bottom of the palm, creating stability for the person to thrive and grow; drawing energy from the Venus mount up into the body, giving nourishment and vitality, and, in particular, establishing a sense of permanence, stability, and security. In medical terms, this line represents homeostasis.

Rather than seeing this line as representing the *length* of life, try to see it as the person's *hold* on life – how realistic, vital, alive, grounded, secure, and stable they are. Strong, clear semicircular earth lines (Figure 10.1) create the physical rhythms of circulating energy, the repetitive patterns of eating, menstruation, sleeping, digestion and excretion, giving one's life rhythm, a cycle of vitality, running through the whole span of the day, the year, the lifetime. Those with a strong line will recover from illness quickly; they have a strong grip on life, they are tenacious and will keep going when any kind of health or life issue interrupts their stability.

Those with weak earth lines (Figure 10.2) find it hard to hold onto stable routines and fixed patterns of life. They tend to panic easily and feel deeply insecure; their energy is uncertain and easily drained, and they lack any sense of permanence. Resilience is difficult to muster to ride life's storms.

The earth line represents the gut, physically. Our gut can send impulses to the brain via nerve fibres, and the earth line is a vital indicator of how our deep intestinal processes are doing. Short, poor-quality earth lines are becoming more common, probably as an effect of children not walking to school and getting little exercise. Also, one must take into account modern diets of highly processed foods, unstable routines, family breakup, and over-stimulation from online activity.

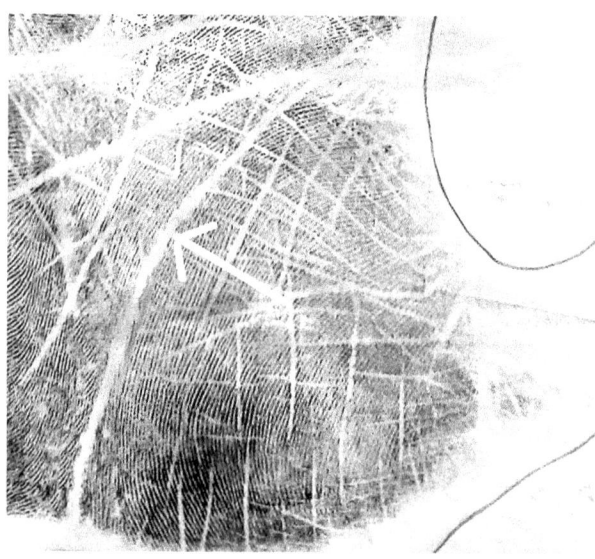

Figure 10.1. Strong earth line.

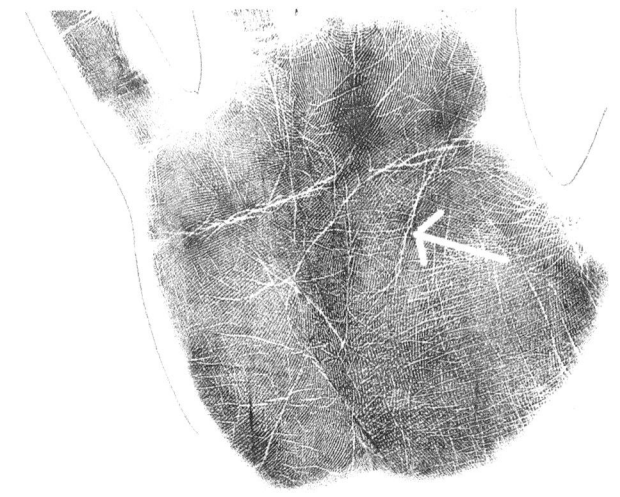

Figure 10.2. Short, weak earth line.

If the earth line is short and feeble, the bearer will have poor assimilation of minerals; there will be insecurity, poor energy, digestive problems, no pattern to diet, activity, or routine; they will lack a sense of permanence. People with poor earth lines lack guts, literally and metaphorically; they cannot dig deep into their resources and are easily panicked by life experiences. Such people often work in realms like complementary therapies, spiritual healing, acting, and the arts. They reach for higher realms to provide a longed-for sense of health and stability. They need security from outside themselves, usually in the form of a steady partner, material wealth, or lots of help and support to keep stable, rather the way a weak shoot will cling to the trunk of an oak to survive. If such a sign is on both hands, they will have had no sense of stability from birth; family life was uncertain, with no rhythm; they are apt to feel easily threatened and unsure of their ground. The same weak line will almost certainly be present on one of the parents' hands.

Irritable bowel, Crohn's disease, and ulcerative colitis are very likely to arise at some point in their lives, and inevitably gut problems will flare up when in crisis. People with such lines have a nervous disposition and cannot digest anything when stressed.

A plus point of a weak earth line, however, is that the person is highly mobile and extremely opportunistic – often people who attain the glittering heights of showbiz or attain great prominence in life do so because their insecurity gives them enormous capacity for social mobility. Despite a nervous gut and digestive issues, they are lightning-quick at adapting to different partners, substitute parents, and new careers, cultures, and countries. This is much easier if the earth line is fragile. To lack a stable lifestyle is useful in unstable, demanding vocations that require you to let go of the rock of home and family and devote everything to a new path.

Babies are usually born with only half an earth line, and only a half-developed gut and digestive system (this is why initially they cannot digest anything other than milk). Within the first 10–15 years of life the earth line develops and lengthens to its full extent, as long as the child is provided with a stable and secure family situation.

It is a good idea for anyone with a weak earth line to have a mineral test to establish which minerals they lack (a weak line assimilates minerals poorly and certain minerals, like magnesium and zinc, are almost always lacking). They should consult a nutritionist and fine-tune their diet to get the nutrients they need. Inevitably the gut biota will need to be supplemented. Rebuilding a weak earth line takes a year or more and requires a totally fixed, stable routine, regular exercise (preferably at the same time each day), the avoidance of stress, and all the herbs, nutrients, and probiotics possible to give the optimum nutrition. They need to make sure to get enough rest, and good sleep is a vital issue. They must learn to relax and be more in touch with their "gut" feelings.

People whose earth lines on both hands are deep, clear, and complete are able to stand on their own two feet and thrive. Such roots deliver abundant nutrients and energy, good vitality, a feeling of being grounded, with a sense of place, good digestion, and internal stability.

Broken earth lines

Clear breaks in any major line are rare. Usually there is an overlap where a second section of the line overlaps the first (Figure 10.3). A seemingly short earth line may be overlapped by a new section of line, very often with a hairline thread connecting the two. Overlapped breaks denote a break in continuity and a major change in life. What is important in these cases is to note the condition and position of the new section of line. If the new overlapping section is strong and well-formed, it's a very positive sign, meaning a person will adapt into new circumstances, and the quality of life, health, and energetic levels will improve. But if the new line is weaker, thinner, and of poorer quality, this could indicate that change will present difficulties and may have detrimental effects on health unless steps are taken. The hangover of traditional predictive palmistry's dictum that a broken earth line (lifeline) foretells an early death means that anyone with a break in the line needs to be reassured that no disaster can come of such signs. They should make sure to have good health always foremost in mind, before all other goals. In particular, they need to live in harmony with the natural rhythms of life without over-reaching themselves in stressful vocations and efforts to feel secure. It is fascinating to see the earth lines of people like farmers and landscape gardeners who must live and work according to nature, the seasons, and natural cycles – they always have amazingly good earth lines.

On the passive hand, a clean break with no overlap in this line (Figure 10.4) indicates a major disturbance in upbringing, usually this is parental divorce, a major move, loss of a family member, or other shock to stability. On the active, a clean break in the line means a dislocation at some point in the rhythm of life in the self-created home, family, or lifestyle. Very often there is an event midlife when a disruption occurs that threatens stability (unless steps are taken to repair the break) and a consequent period of exhaustion and vulnerability to illness. Timing is vague and difficult to judge on the lines, but on female hands most

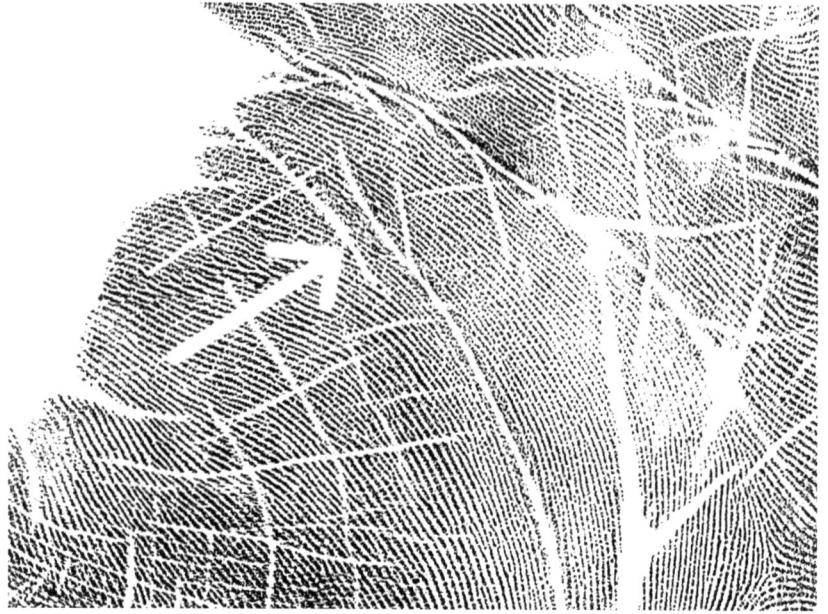

Figure 10.3. Broken earth line with overlap.

breaks occur around two thirds of the way down and coincide with the menopause.

A break in a person's active earth line means expectations of health, place, and home are never quite fulfilled, and life is a process of striving to get the resources they feel they need. Very often this manifests as a need to constantly re-decorate the home, earn more money, or to start new health diet and exercise regimes that never quite fill the vacancy they feel in themselves. If the line is of good quality despite the break, there is a good chance it can form "bridge lines" over the break and become whole when a fixed, stable, and natural regimen is adapted. It is also important to make the person understand that life is full of ups and downs, and we all have to face old age, frailty, and a letting-go eventually. In particular they need to sleep better and get enough rest.

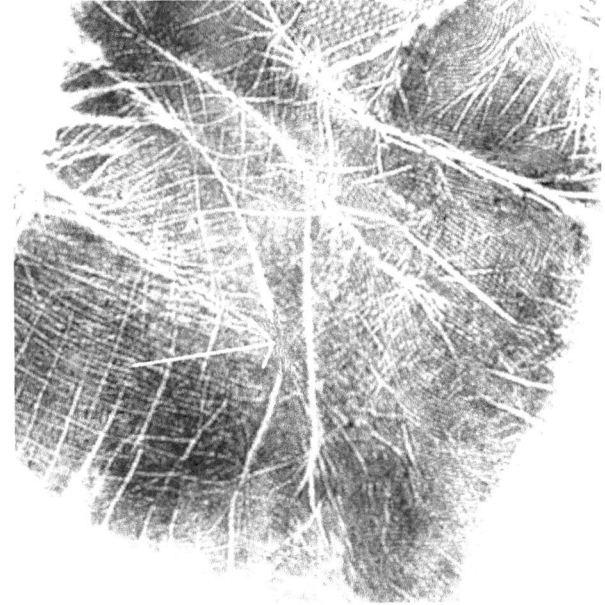

Figure 10.4. A break in the earth line with no overlap.

Missing base of the earth line

Where just the very base of the earth line is missing (Figure 10.5) on the passive hand, it's because the family was never fixed in one place, continually uprooted or changed cultures. This is very common on first-generation immigrants and the children of highly mobile parents. On the active hand it shows someone who functions well in terms of health and stability (assuming the rest of the line is of good quality) but who never really has a sense of belonging anywhere. The missing base means never being fixed to a particular home or country. Someone with a missing base section doesn't know where they stand in life; they are usually clumsy, having poor balance and problems with feet and knees. They are prone to lofty, ungrounded lifestyles, values,

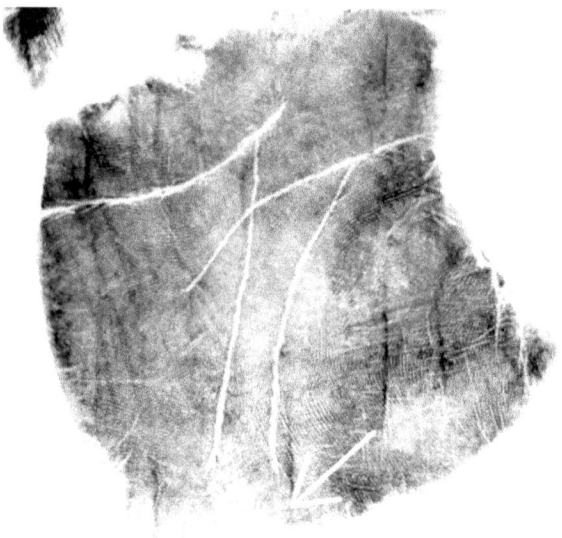

Figure 10.5. Earth line with missing base section.

and schemes and are in danger of ignoring practical health advice. Very often the missing section creates a fastidious terror of germs, dirt, and bacteria. The last part of the line relates to the sphincter and often indicates haemorrhoids, fissures, or tears in this area.

An earth line made up of tiny islands is like a root saturated with water: it shows a person bogged down by family and health issues with highs and lows of vitality. Such people often have a leaky gut and love comfort foods and taking frequent baths.

A large island on the earth line (Figure 10.6) is a rare sign and is a big warning: if on both hands, they will usually appear near the base of the line and indicate a late-onset period of immobility and some kind of life sapping condition. When seen on the active hand, appropriate action needs to be taken: a thorough health scan and lifestyle re think is needed. The line may well then mend itself before there is any danger.

THE MAJOR EARTH LINE 75

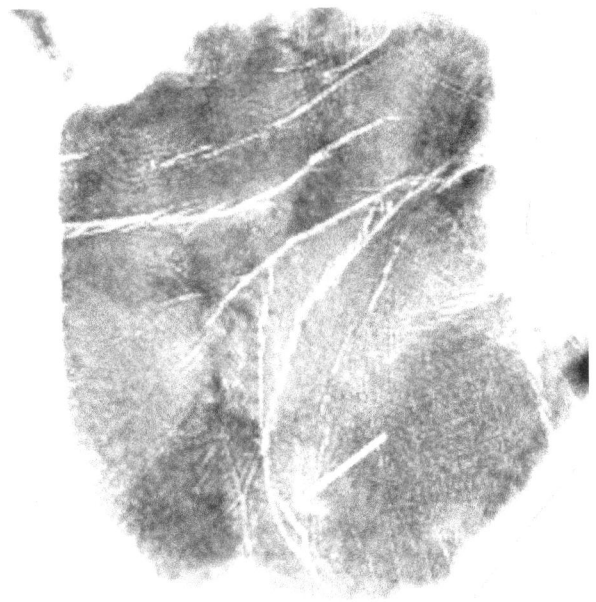

Figure 10.6. Large island on the earth line.

A very thick, trough-like earth line looks amazingly strong and full of vitality but needs to be examined carefully. If the line is clear and well formed, this is an excellent sign. However, if the line is very thick, with an eroded, fading quality at the edges, it can show a sluggish, clogged intestine and a poor diet. Those blessed with amazingly strong, deep, clear earth lines all too often take their fabulous constitution for granted. They may well survive with no ill effects on a junk food diet until deep into their fifties when the edges of the earth line starts to crumble away and health issues catch up with them (Figure 10.7).

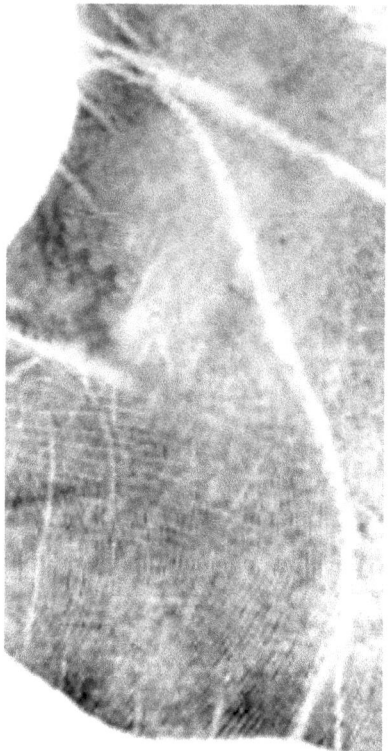

Figure 10.7. Note the nibbled edges to this earth line – this is on the hand of a drummer in a rock band who lives on crisps and pizza.

The sweep of the earth line

The natural shape of the earth line is a semicircle around the thumb mount. If we extend the metaphor of the root, we can see the thumb ball is the mound of fertile earth the root draws its nutrients from. On around 5% of palms, the earth line and mount bulges much further out than normal, beyond the centre of the palm. It shows physical prowess, life force in abundance, and tremendous vitality – the drive to get really stuck into anything. Whenever you see a wide-swept line, it guarantees an adventurous soul with abundant drive and ample physical resources – it's common on performers and sportspeople (Figure 10.8).

On 2% of palms, the earth line is confined to a narrow semicircle, staying very close to the thumb (Figure 10.9). This will be accompanied by a flat, soft thumb ball. It shows timidity and restraint. Such a line denotes someone who stays indoors and close to home. It is common on those with anxieties about travel, risk, and open spaces. They should be careful not to tax themselves too much and to avoid stressful and demanding vocations. The mount and line can be strengthened by gentle exercise, like yoga.

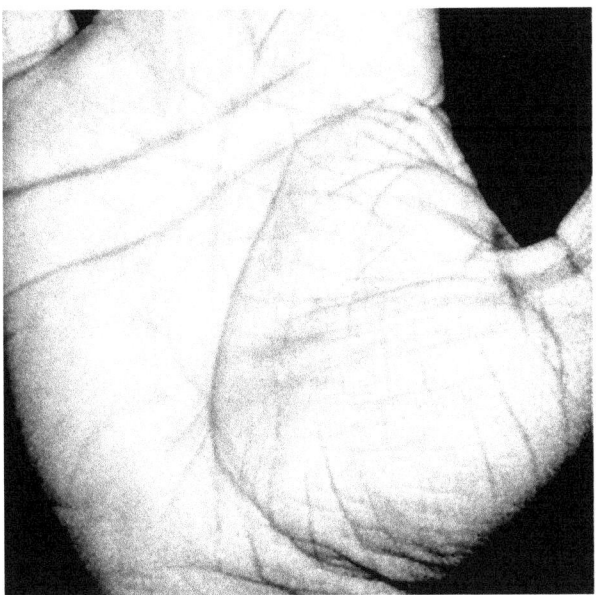

Figure 10.8. Wide sweep to earth line on an Olympic fencing champion.

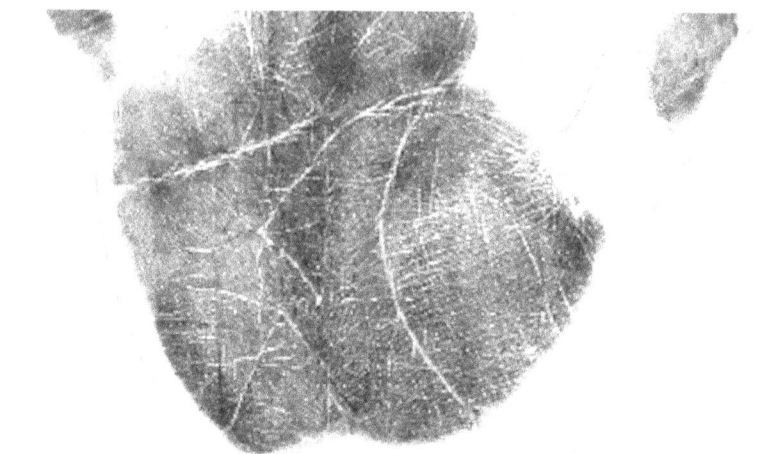

Figure 10.9. Narrow sweep to earth line.

Always remember: in the passive hand, a break, an island, or a short line indicates a pattern inherited from parental background and childhood. If this is not replicated on the active hand, this problem or condition is unlikely to occur. It is like a shadow that may come to light if the person's lifestyle is seriously unhealthy – like an unwelcome visitor lurking in the shadows.

11

The major air line

The meaning, metaphor, and nature of the air line

The air line (traditionally called the head line) is a key aspect to understanding a person's personality, as it shows the nature of their thinking process. Whether we think independently, logically, symbolically, or objectively, is to a great extent what make us ourselves. People with very different air lines are on different wavelengths: they perceive the world in differing ways. Strong, deep, red air lines make for strongly held views and forceful characters; weak, fragmented air lines are found on more fragile-minded and ambivalent individuals.

The metaphor for this line is a light beam. Keep this in mind, as it will be extremely useful in your understanding of this line. Notice how often we use this metaphor for mental qualities: "she's a bright spark", "it came in a flash". Indeed, we say that gaining wisdom is the process of becoming enlightened. Physically, the air line rules the solar plexus, and affects breathing, concentration, mental stability, clarity, and eyesight.

Difficult beginnings

The first section beneath the index is very indicative of how bold or timid we are. If the line is joined to the earth line for a long way (Figure 11.1), not breaking free until almost beneath the middle finger, it indicates one of life's late developers. This is a sign of someone who cannot think independently and only broke free of dominating parents or traditional beliefs mid-life. It is common on those who hyperventilate under stress and who have been brought up in a very restrictive religious or military setting.

If the line is beginning widely separated from the earth line (Figure 11.2), this is the totally opposite scenario. This indicates abundant confidence, independence, sense of adventure, and someone with a mind free of parental values. If on the passive hand, this could be seen as a sign of recklessness (with a greater risk from accidents) when young.

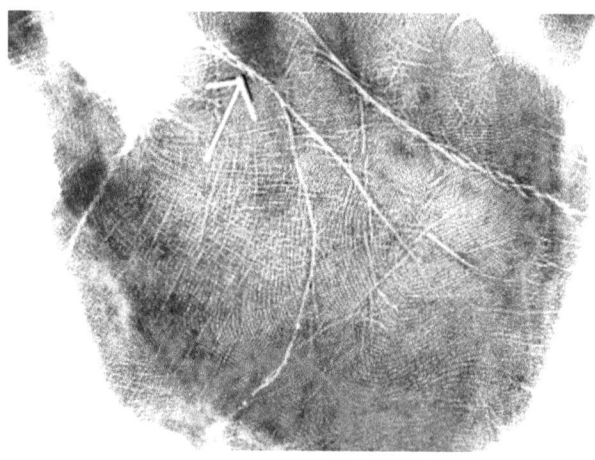

Figure 11.1. Joined air and earth lines.

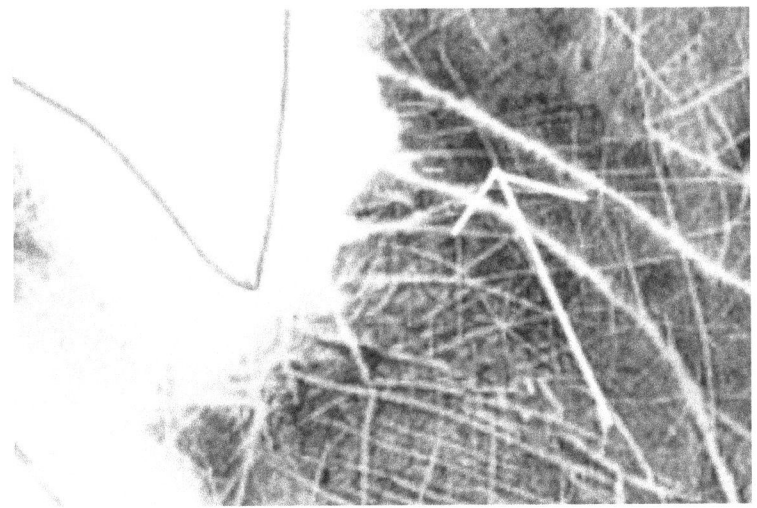

Figure 11.2. Separate air and earth lines.

Sinus troubles, excess mucus, snoring, and ear, nose, and throat issues are indicated if the first section of the air line is a mess of scribbly lines or has an island on the active hand (Figure 11.3). If on the passive hand (much more common), this is an underlying childhood issue.

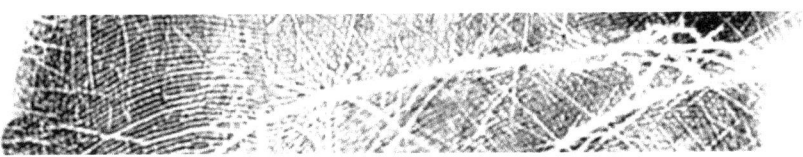

Figure 11.3. Messy beginning of an air line.

The long and the short of it: the length of the air line

The longer this line extends across the palm, the further, mentally, one illuminates the darkness of possibility and more that needs to be taken into consideration in any decision. Long lines (ending under the little finger) have a long thinking process. They take a long view, they look a long way ahead, and are highly philosophical. Short lines (ending under the middle digit) illuminate their immediate circumstances and are concerned only with enacting ideas. A line ending under the ring digit is of average length. It is fascinating that long lines tend to eventually develop long-sightedness, and short ones, near-sightedness; this is not guaranteed, but can often become an issue after the age of 50.

A short air line (Figure 11.4) sees a small picture and is more immediate and focused on what is before them, the way a bright desk lamp illuminates only what is on the table. Contrary to what you might expect, those with short air lines (if clear and well

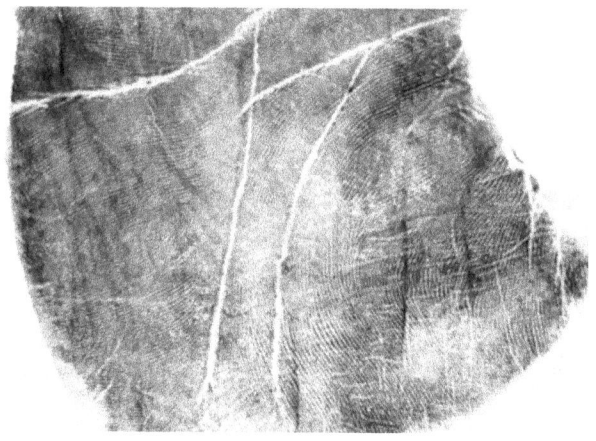

Figure 11.4. Short air line.

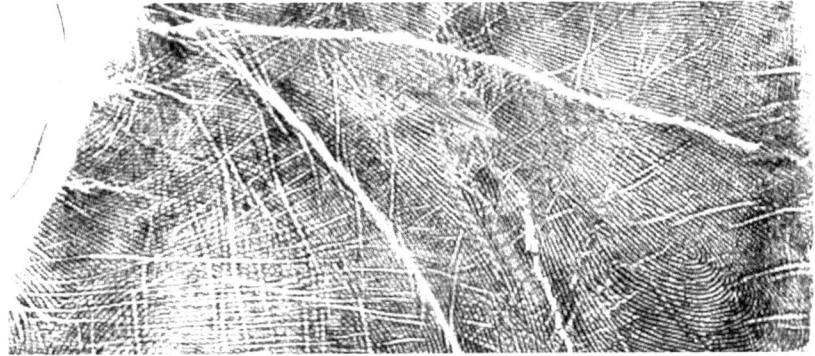

Figure 11.5.   Long air line.

formed) are extremely focused, highly productive, and amazingly effective people. They have no distractions, no philosophy, no speculating over future outcomes. They put all their mental energy into getting things done and applying their minds to real-world situations. They are, however, unable to see a broader view, and so this is a strong indication of high stress levels and the possibility of burnout. (Other signs in the hand will affirm or contradict this in a later chapter on signs of stress.)

People who have long, clear air lines (Figure 11.5) are philosophical, curious, speculative, and analytical. Their long torch-beam minds look into many possible outcomes and are much less likely to fall victim to stress via short-sighted plans, as there is always a wider perspective.

Sydney lines

A line that continues straight across the hand to touch the other side is known as a Sydney line (Figure 11.6) – as it was first investigated and explained by palmist Andrew Fitzherbert in Sydney, Australia. It crosses the palm completely and creates a compulsive thought process. All complete crossing major lines in the hand give an immense strength and present an outer calm while concealing a brittle, fixed nature. All crossing lines create a compulsion.

Sydney lines have a tough quality, mentally. Though outwardly serene, their deeper selves are unavailable. They can easily ignore the demands of the body and become constipated, sleepless, or unable to eat. Notoriously, Sydney-lined people are very hard on themselves and rarely seek help, no matter what pain or illness besets them. Usually they are thin and edgy but outwardly in control, particularly in difficult and dangerous situations. Sydney air line people think obsessively, and this is linked to high intelligence but also to various childhood learning and behavioural difficulties and certain blood conditions. If on the passive hand, dyslexia is strongly suggested, as well as ADHD and obsessive behaviour. There is a higher risk of childhood leukaemia.

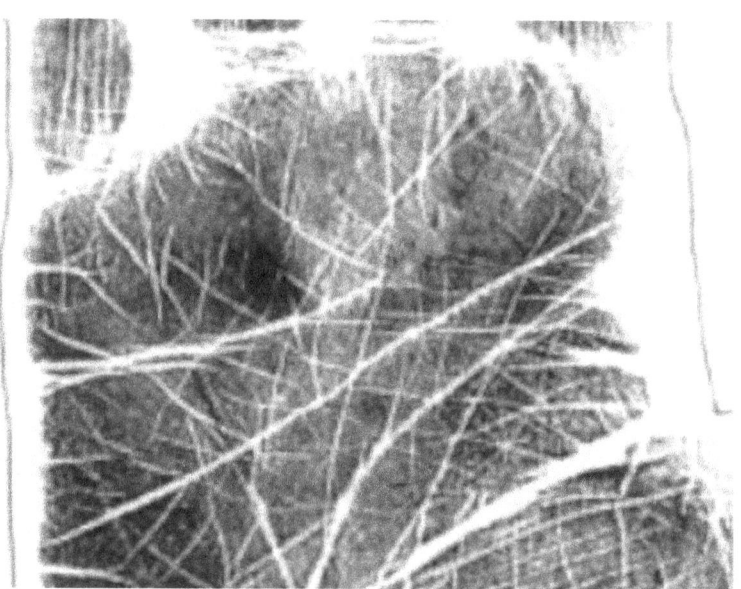

Figure 11.6. Sydney line.

Very often where there is a Sydney line in both hands, childhood dyslexia and other issues are eventually overcome, and a late-developing prodigy with tremendous strength of mind emerges. Childhood and early adulthood, though, may have shown little promise. The bearer of such a line often eventually learns to use their obsessive thinking process to achieve great things. It is speculated that the complete crossing line develops because of a need to be constantly vigilant, as if the light beam of the mind is ever watchful because of difficulties within the home environment. In a small number of cases this triggers white blood cells to be overproduced, as there is a higher incidence of childhood leukaemia and sickle cell anaemia, as well as ventricular septal defect (hole in the heart, present at birth) (Bhanu, "Simian Crease [Sydney line] in Man"). This is obviously only a statistical higher incidence of such conditions, but the risk is heightened if accompanied by a raised axial triradius.

Air line quality: clear or cloudy?

Always check the clarity of the air line – if the light beam is unclear, broken up, full of little islands, or crossed by multiple little lines (Figure 11.7), the person cannot see clearly, their mental picture is incoherent, and health issues are likely in the very long term. No matter how long the line, conceptually, they are in a mental fog of stress and distraction. Poor-quality lines are found on highly frazzled people lacking a clear sense of their own judgement. Brain fog, depression, forgetfulness, exhaustion, vision problems, and chest infections are much more common in those with weak air lines. A chain of small islands on this line warns against overtaxing one's mental reserves, so they should always be advised to not, for example, take on a maths degree while raising two children. Any serious mental undertaking is creating more vulnerability to health troubles.

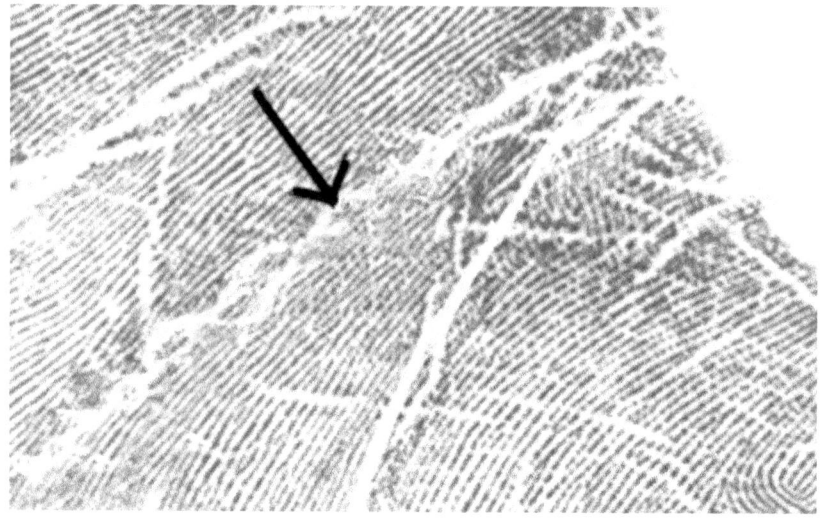

Figure 11.7. Frazzled air line.

Any large island on the air line (Figure 11.8) is always a sign of stress. An island is like a bubble of mental energy circulating around and around without resolution. It indicates someone with a "short circuit" in their mental attitude they cannot see a way out of. An island in a line splits the flow of energy, so susceptibility to bronchial, breathing, and respiratory issues is indicated. Islands mark mentally stressful points in life, where the mind distorts an issue out of proportion. It is possible that a mineral imbalance could be an underlying factor. Diet might be investigated, as the sodium/potassium balance in the body may be out of kilter.

Check which finger an island is found under to reveal something of the cause. An island under the index finger relates to problems in ambition, self-belief, control, and sense of self; under the middle finger: marriage, money, social obligations, security or work; under the ring finger: looks, image, creativity, self-expression; under the little finger: ideas, finance, business, communication, or sex. Air line islands require serious strate-

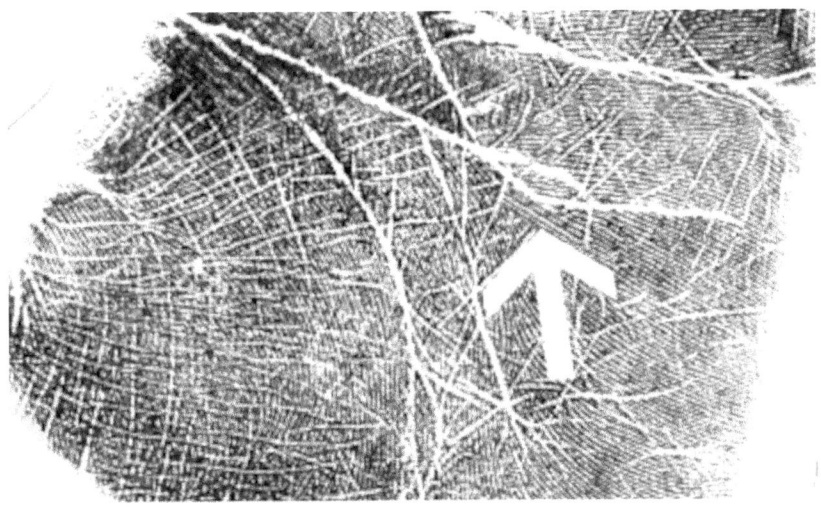

Figure 11.8. Large island on air line.

gies to heal, so objective third-party guidance is always needed to resolve the issue. Multiple sclerosis, nervous tics, dementia, periods of mental breakdown, and nervous complaints have been linked to large islands in the air line.

Bent or straight? The path of the air line

Where the air line is straight, moving horizontally across the palm, the mind processes ideas in a logical, straight-line manner – direct, factual, evidence-based, objective: the truth is all that matters. The straight-line mind avoids dipping deep into the subconscious area of the palm (the quadrant that sits in the lower part of the palm opposite the thumb ball). Mental projections are of the proven, logical world. If they daydream, it's about real people and actual life events, potential or past. Straight air lines are highly stable psychologically. They can be blunt – things are black-and-white, wrong or right; they will not be persuaded without reference to facts, statistics, and evidence.

Curved air lines (Figure 11.9) are subjective and see things personally. The world takes on different clothes according to the mood they are in, their past experiences, their own reflections. They are more buried within themselves, more introverted and more inclined to be artistic and intuitive. Their perceptions are more coloured, and the cold facts don't impress them at all. Where straight, long air lines enjoy debate and argument; curved lines do not.

If the air line is *very* bent, it shows a withdrawal psychologically into the inner realm; sometimes extremely deep and introspective. A very bent air line person will often be unable to tell you exactly where they go in their own minds and will need to be quiet, alone, and withdrawn for long periods of time. Deep plunging air lines like half-light, shadows, and dark, secret spaces. On the passive hand, this is a sure sign of a solitary childhood, inner withdrawal, and general introversion. Bent air lines are less stable in their mindsets than straight ones. Periods of depression are

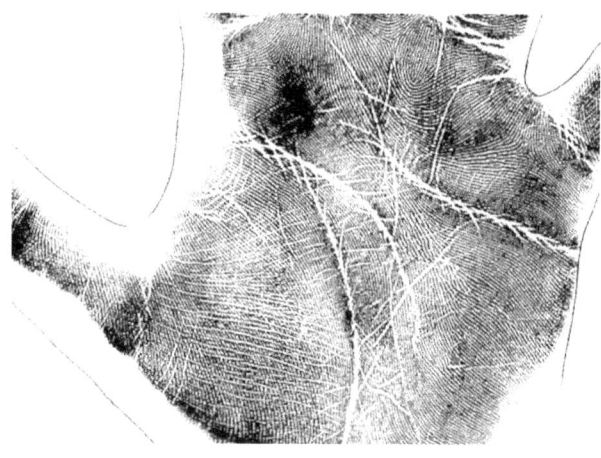

Figure 11.9.   Bent air line.

much more likely with this pattern. The long bent line is common on people who literally or metaphorically burrow into the mind's dark places: conspiracy theorists, writers, researchers, poets, artists, and psychoanalysts. The bent air line is much more common on those with psychosomatic illnesses, bipolar episodes, schizophrenia, and antisocial behaviour.

Change and new directions

It is important to note that the air line is one of the quickest to change; a person with a chaotic line needs to be advised to develop concentration: a still point in the mind through the practice of mindfulness and fixed focus. They must avoid stress at all costs. Working in nature in a physical way has a remarkably good effect on a disturbed air line, bringing clarity and coherence. The air line will often lengthen when a broad holistic subject is studied, such as comparative philosophy (Figures 11.10 and 11.11).

Breaks in the air line

Where the air line is in two sections (Figure 11.12), it illustrates a sort of dual personality, where a person can shift between two perspectives, personalities, and outlooks. This is a rare marking. If on the active hand, it always points to a possible midlife crisis and subsequent change in that person's mindset. On the passive hand, it indicates a shift in educational development and points to some kind of life change. Whenever you see an air line in two sections, understand the person will always be striving to get "get to the other side". This means they are never satisfied with the way things are and want to extend themselves to learn new skills,

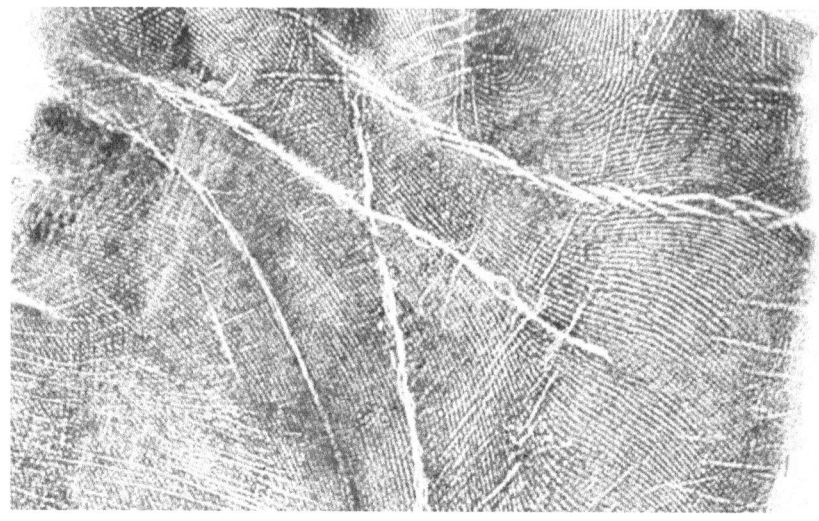

Figure 11.10. Before a yoga teacher training course.

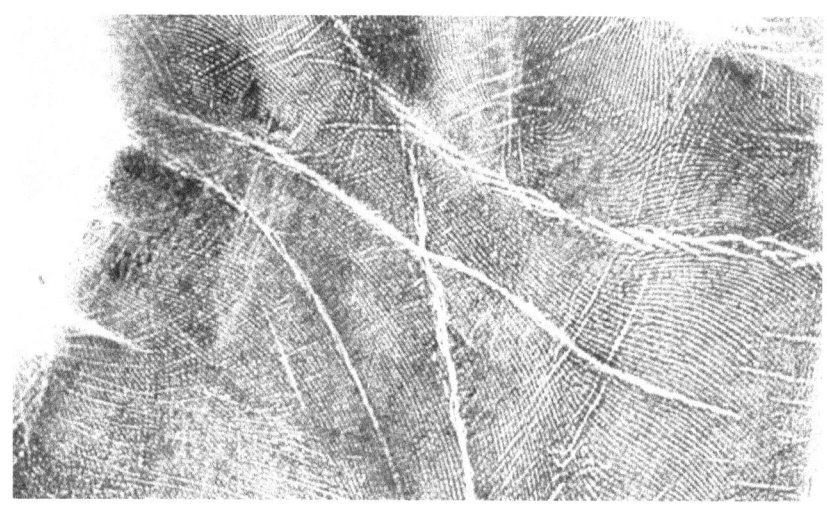

Figure 11.11. Air line after a year of yoga training.

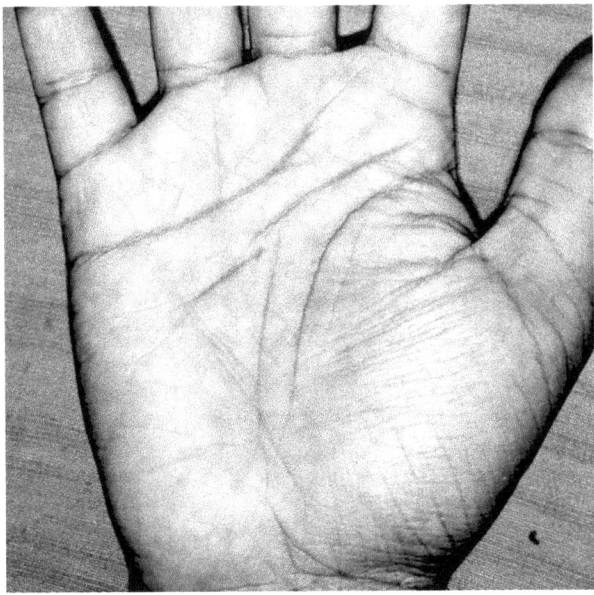

Figure 11.12. An air line in two sections.

acquire a new perspective, have a different vision (the other section of the line). This is a classic "grass is always greener" syndrome. It often leads to a person over-extending themselves, to dissatisfaction with the way things are. It can lead to great disappointment if not explained to the bearer of this marking.

Single transverse palmar crease

Sometimes (in around 1% of people), the air and water lines are united in a single crease, known as a single transverse palmar crease (Figure 11.13).

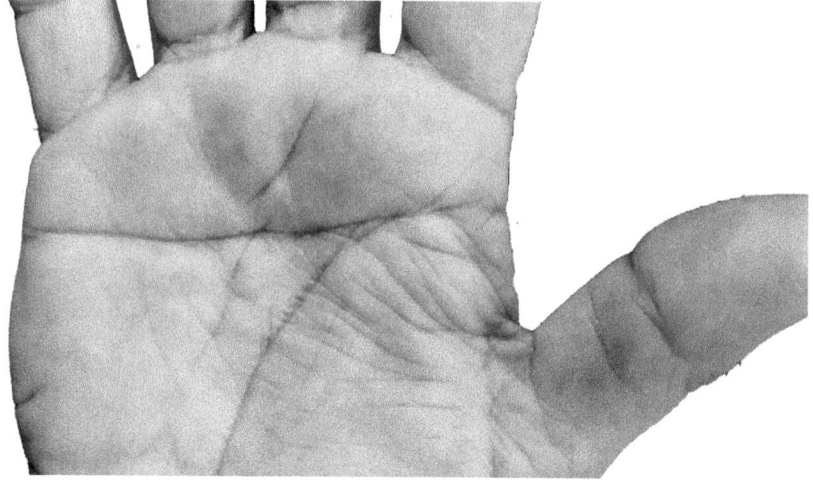

Figure 11.13. Single transverse palmar crease.

This is the sign of an intense, obsessive personality. Single-transverse- palmar folk are like a repressed, silently raging storm; thought and feeling are synonymous. They appear rock-steady: all their emotional and intellectual energy is internalised. They put all their feelings and ideas into their goals in a relentless, single-minded manner. This can, of course, lead to great achievements, and, indeed, it's disproportionately found on highly successful people, particularly in fields where absolute dedication is necessary: professional athletes, intellectuals, movie stars, meticulous, dedicated researchers, self-made business magnates – the single transverse palmar crease line is found on over 14% of such individuals.

As the water and air lines are running together, they tend to be emotionally and psychologically closed, with one-track minds, unable to be frivolous or jump from one subject to another. They find it difficult to relax and are usually either extremely charming social operators or highly withdrawn, reticent and awkward socially. Single-transverse- palmar-crease-lined folk tend to get stuck in patterns – never letting go of their thesis, agenda, goal, business plan, design, family issue, or ex-partner. They find it extremely difficult to see another's viewpoint and stick to their beliefs, come what may. Once possessed of a feeling or idea, they rarely let go of it.

The most common manifestation of the single transverse palmar crease line is in Downs syndrome – some 60% of them have this on either or both palms). This is accompanied by a variety of other palm markers (as mentioned in the Introduction), including a palm with very few lines; unnaturally short digits, with all fingers bearing loop fingerprints that lift to a point only half way up the fingertips; a raised axial triradius; and a little finger with only two phalanges.

The single transverse palmar crease line is linked to a number of childhood chromosome abnormalities, including fetal alcohol syndrome, cri du chat syndrome, Klinefelter syndrome, Wolf-Hirschhorn Syndrome, Noonan syndrome, Patau syndrome, Edward's syndrome and Aarskog-Scott syndrome. Frightening though these issues are, remember that the vast majority of people with a single transverse palmar crease line will not have these issues. However, it's fair to say that they are likely to be much more driven, intense, and repressed than the general population, and this is a marker for a tendency towards aggression, anger, and obstinacy, as well as difficulties in intimate relationships that can negatively impact their personal and professional lives. They are also more prone to hypertension, respiratory issues, cardiovascular diseases, and reproductive system issues.

Sources

Bhanu, V. "Simian crease in man: Some methodological considerations." *Journal of Human Evolution*, Vol. 2, No. 2 (1973): 153–160.

JAMA. "The hand and cardiovascular disease." *Journal of the American Medical Association*, Vol. 154, No. 6 (1994): 508.

Rook, L. W. "Biomarkers of mental illness and the human hand: A systematic review." *European Journal of Psychiatry*, Vol. 36, No. 2 (2022): 77–93.

Shamai-Lubovitz, O., Trattner, A., Katznelson, M. B., & Sandbank, M. "Dermatoglyphics in Darier's disease." *International Journal of Dermatology*, Vol. 33, No. 9 (1994): 626–627.

12

The water line

The meaning, metaphor, and nature of the water line

The water line has the easiest metaphor to imagine, as it's visualised as the river of emotional responses. Its course begins at the palm edge under the little finger, to end somewhere in the area between the index and middle digits. A long line would end under the index finger and a short one under the middle digit.

This line is an indicator of our emotional flow, the way one reacts to a painting, a piece of music, the cry of a child; it's not simply about our relationships. In many ways, the water line is about how rich, joyous, open, connected, and moved we are to the stream of life.

See this line as the river of feeling that transports us emotionally. If the line is deep and strong, the river sweeps us along. A moving film or uplifting section of music will be impossible to ignore: involuntarily, the heart will move in the chest, one is compelled to respond. If the line's weak and broken, the tune or film will leave a person cold. The depth of the line reflects the depth of feeling: a deep, red line reflects powerful passions, whereas a shallow line is more reticent.

Physically, the line rules the heart organ for the first third of its length, and its overall flow indicates the circulation, the condition of the blood vessels, as well as the movement of synovial and lymphatic fluid. The deeper and stronger the line, the more powerful the bodily fluids and passions flow.

Water line quality

The quality of the water line is all about how free the flow of the emotions is. Obviously, if the line's scratchy and full of breaks, the stream of empathy and feeling is more a tangled ditch than a fast-flowing river (Figure 12.1). This shows poor circulation, varicose veins, cold hands and feet, lymphatic issues, a sense of isolation and disconnection. Many weak water line people have a tendency to indulge in excess alcohol to free up the emotions and "let go". It is hard to express oneself in fun activities – art, music,

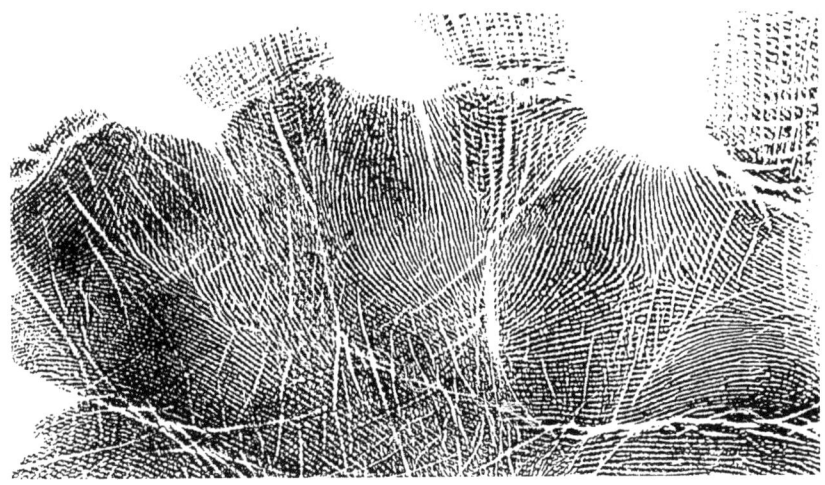

Figure 12.1. Weak, poor-quality water line.

dance – and be joyful if the line is poor. Scratchy water lines lack the enthusiasm for team sports, communal activities and the arts, though they are strongly represented in commercial cold-blooded, modern art, without heart or feeling. Perversely, a poor-quality water line person is more likely to hold onto a relationship than a strong water line one: they more easily feel cut off from others – hence the need to stay in an (often difficult) partnership. Weak, scratchy heart lines don't want risks in relationships and find it hard to trust their feelings.

Dental problems, gum disease, and tooth decay are indicated where the water line is poor in quality. Research has established links between gum issues (periodontal disease) and a higher risk of stroke or other serious cardiovascular event. Poor circulation is always indicated by a poor-quality line, particularly if the hands feel cold at room temperature.

Large islands or breaks on this line (Figure 12.2) under the ring finger have been linked to heart events – this part of the line rules that organ. These are a clear warning to have regular heart and blood-pressure checks, and to take herbs and supplemental support as well as to exercise and maintain a low-cholesterol diet. This is especially true if the triradius is higher than average and if there are many whorls present on the fingertips.

Lots of fine, hair-like lines crossing the water line (Figure 12.3) have been linked to heart arrhythmia and palpitations: it's as if the river emotion is turbulent and is endlessly caught up in cross-currents.

A series of red dots on the water line (Figure 12.4) have been observed where there is a build-up of cholesterol: this is a worrying sign of possible heart events.

Where there is a deep, strong, water line, a person cannot *help* feeling, connecting with, and responding to people, art, music, play, children, and spiritual impulses. They simply *must* be in love and strongly connected or would rather not be in a relationship at all. They will be more inclined to take emotive leaps, to trust their feelings, and to throw themselves into communal and caring activities.

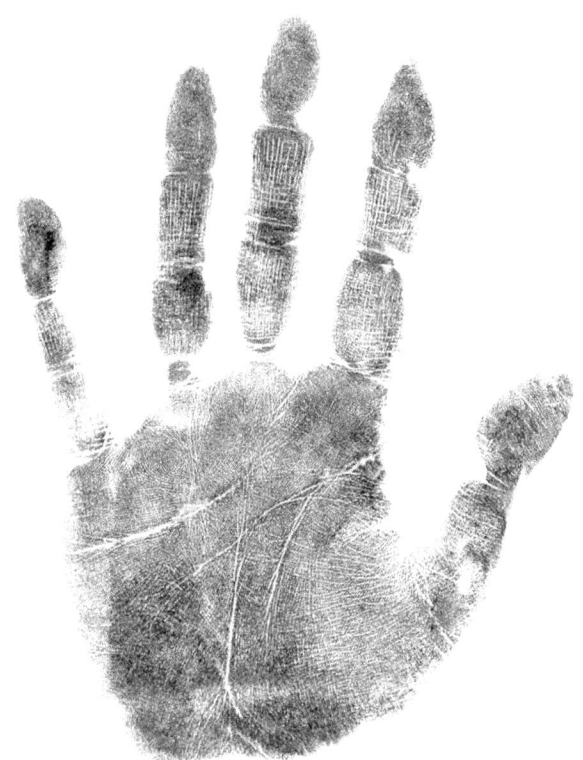

Figure 12.2. Island on water line beneath ring digit.

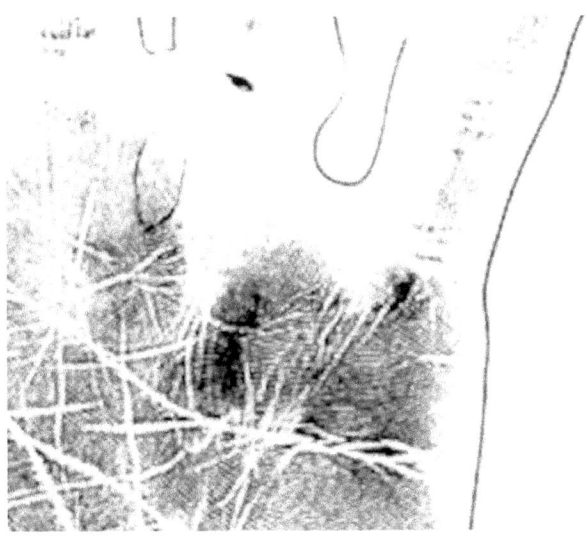

Figure 12.3. Water line with lots of crossing lines.

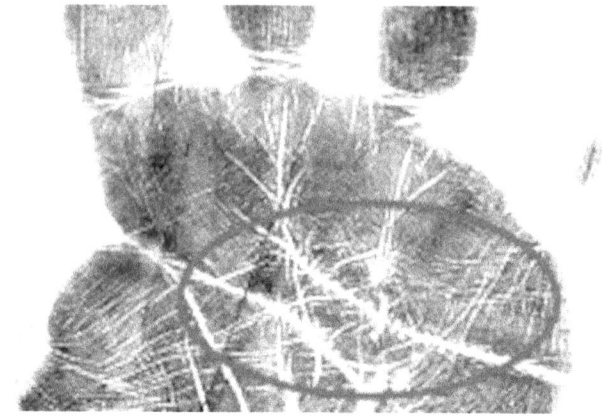

Figure 12.4. Water line with multiple dots along its length.

Straight or curved?

A curved water line (like the one in Figure 12.5) that rises to end near the top edge of the palm, is like a fountain: expressive, romantic, and idealistic. See the raised ending as spring, breaking

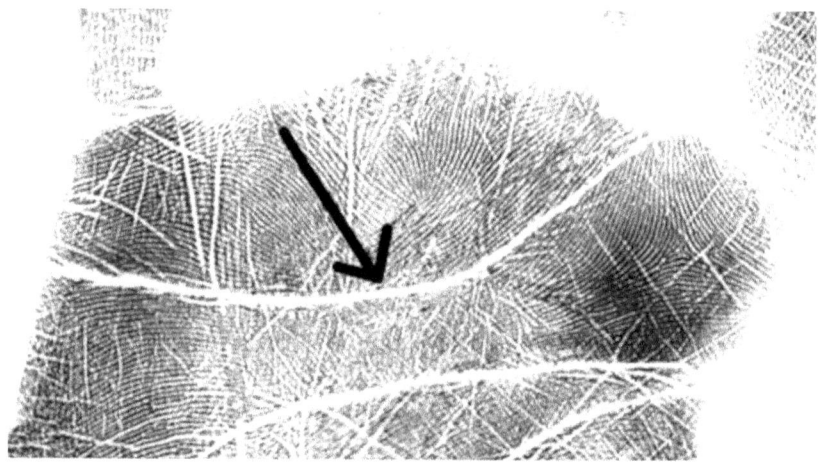

Figure 12.5. Strong clear water line.

the surface, expressing a spray of emotion, idealism, effusiveness, and romanticism. Curved-line people are expressive, and their feelings gush to the surface – this is considered (as long as the line is clear and strong) as the healthiest ideal for this line, though it's found only on around 25% of hands.

A straight water line (Figure 12.6), however, is more direct and less expressive. Straight lines are more likely to buy a partner a present or do something practical than spray the partner with expressions of adoration. Straight lines are more pragmatic, more level in their affections, and less geared to one particular partner or love object. They are also much more repressed emotively. Straight heart lines that are broken or full of islands indicate issues with the emotional and arterial flow and someone holding feelings in check. They can point to problems with peripheral blood circulation and consequent possibility of depression.

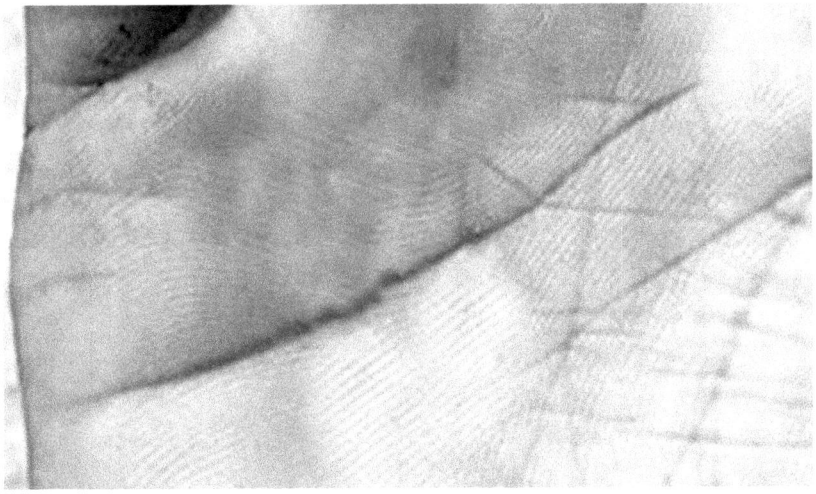

Figure 12.6. Straight water line.

The length of the water line

A short line will end under or before the middle finger (Figure 12.7). This indicates the breadth of emotions doesn't extend very far. The person cannot empathise with anyone outside their immediate family. They will be blunt, unsentimental, and maybe somewhat hard-hearted. If found short, poor in quality, and straight, with coarse skin, it can be the sign of a sociopath, who shuns the company of others and relates only to dogs, plants, and siblings. In the long term, this indicates, medically, hardening of the arteries, high cholesterol, and angina.

Long lines, which end under the index finger (Figure 12.8) indicate people who have a lot of friends; they extend their emotional drive into the wider world, a lot of people and more distant relationships. It is the sign of a carer: a sympathetic and emphatic person. Long-water-lined people tend to be diplomatic and careful not to offend others: often they are carers, therapists, nurses, and other empathic souls.

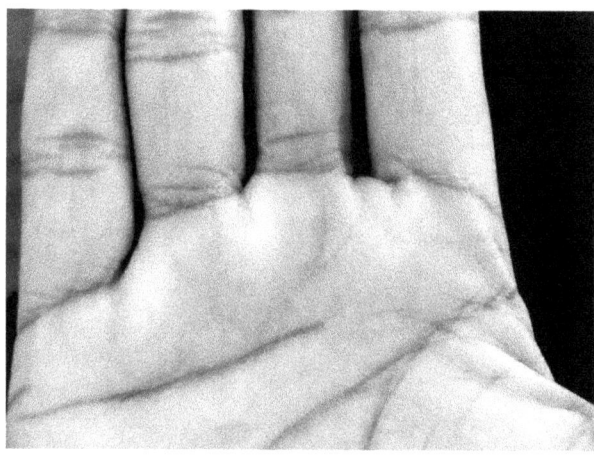

Figure 12.7. Short water line.

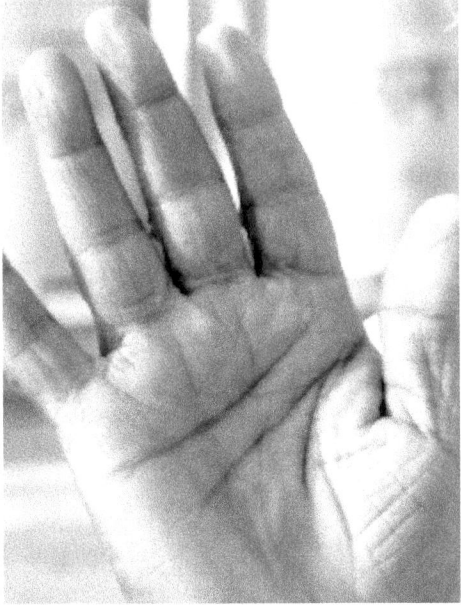

Figure 12.8. Long water line.

In full flood: complete crossing water lines

Where the water line crosses the palm completely from side to side (Figure 12.9), it creates an obsessive kindness: it's not possible for them to be unresponsive emotively. All complete crossing lines create obsessive behaviour. Though compassionate and caring souls, people with this sign simply cannot say "no".

Very long lines are extremely common on all sorts of therapists and professional carers. As the line is flat, not curving to a more abstract ideal, they demonstrate emotions practically. Surprisingly, such people are often poor at one-to-one relationships, despite their compassionate natures. A torrent of emotion floods across

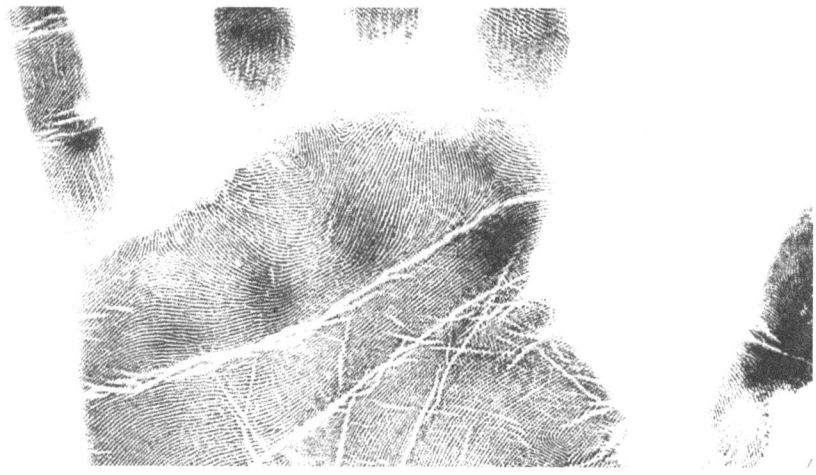

Figure 12.9. Complete crossing water line.

the hand, blocking the demonstrative process and rendering them repressive and unlikely to whisper words of love – yet they are full of caring devotion. Often the demands of others put a great strain on personal relationships. Reynaud's disease and various other circulatory disorders are linked to this sign. The heart organ itself is not affected, but this pattern puts a strain on the movement and pressure within the blood vessels.

If the line is very deep and red and is the strongest major line, and if the hand is warm even on a cool day, it's a sign of high blood pressure. It is as if the water of emotions (and blood supply) is in full flood and under pressure.

High emotions

If the water line ends at the base of the index finger (Figure 12.10), this is rare and creates emotional idealism. This sign means that they will put their partners on a pedestal and hold them to the highest standards. It is hard for them to be satisfied with the merely mortal – their expectations are impossible to live up to. It can create perfectionism in matters of romance and love, and it's crucial that this is pointed out to the bearer. This pattern is linked to over-excitement, artistic and romantic perfectionism, and mania.

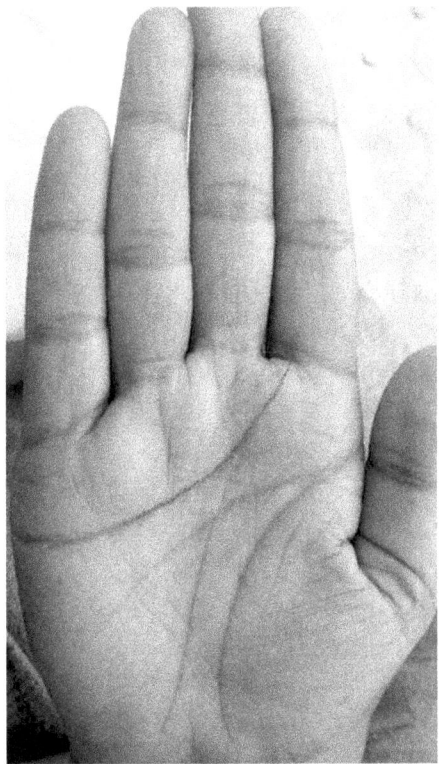

Figure 12.10. Water line with idealistic ending under index digit.

Dropped endings

The opposite pattern, where the end of the water line drops downward to touch the earth line or comes close to it (Figure 12.11), shows an obsession with the parents, the past, and with childhood. On the passive hand, this ending indicates a strong connection to parents – indeed, someone who cannot let go of their parents and family. On the active hand, this signals a person who needs lots of emotional support and proof of commitment; they are likely to be sentimental, dwelling on the past, and hoarding mementoes. It can be a sign of jealousy and fear of emotive display. It is often linked to holding on to sadness and emotional losses. Many hand readers have noticed a link between this sign and diabetes mellitus.

Lying low

Occasionally, you will find a water line that is very low-set in the palm (Figure 12.12). This is a sign of a hidden, cautious emotional pattern – someone who is reluctant to commit themselves emotionally and who hides their deeper feelings. This person is very hard to know well, and who shows themselves only when very sure of the trust of another. Individuals with low-set lines love exercise and physical movement, as it's a way for them to release emotion. Though this line can appear problematic, it has not been proven to have any medical implications, except low blood pressure.

THE WATER LINE

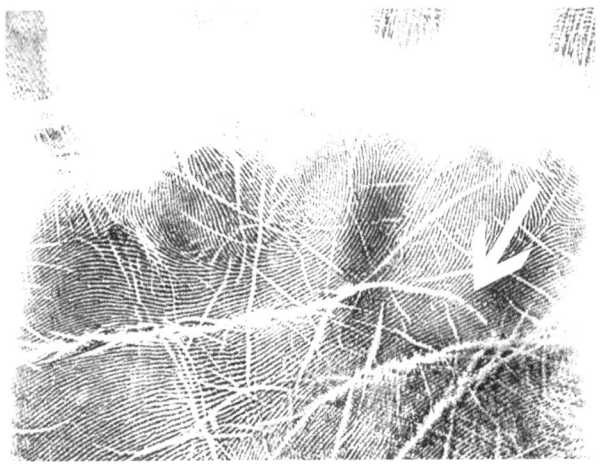

Figure 12.11. Dropped ending to the water line.

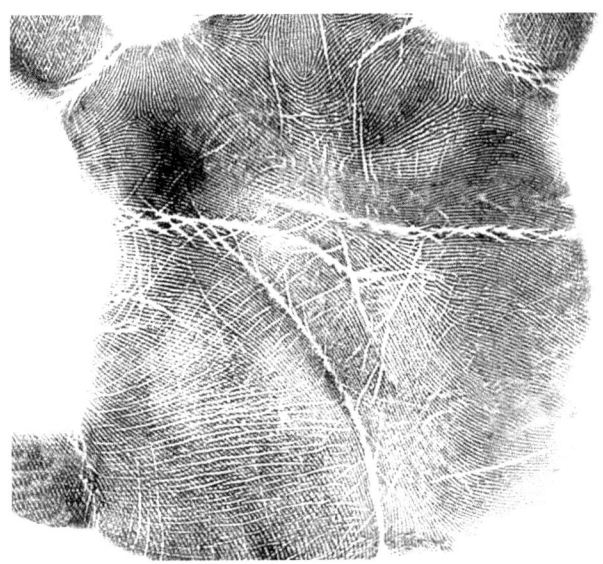

Figure 12.12. Low set water line.

Broken water lines

In the rare case when the water line fractures (Figure 12.13), it signifies a break in a person's emotional life, where the capacity to feel is lost. On the passive hand it's likely they underwent an emotional shock of some kind, within the family set-up. As with all markings, if not replicated on the active hand, there are unlikely to be any health consequences. If the break doesn't occur under the ring finger, the issue will not affect the heart organ itself and is much more likely to indicate some kind of shift in emotional attitudes and shock to the emotions that will affect health to some degree and, in particular, circulation.

All breaks indicate a shift of expression and moving to another level of feeling. A hard knot of skin that seems to almost erase the water line under the ring finger is indicative of heart organ issues. Regular heart and circulatory checks are recommended with any water line with a clean break (except around the last part of

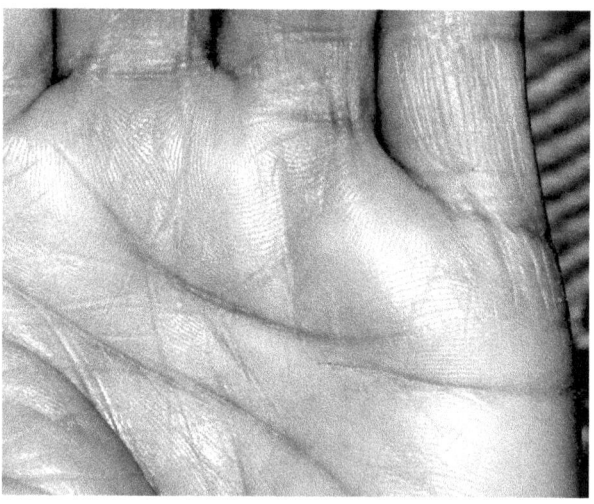

Figure 12.13. Broken water line.

the line near the join of the index and middle finger: this is of no health consequence).

Going with the flow

It is enormously important to encourage to all those with poor water lines, whether broken, erased, with an island, scratchy, or short, to develop their emotional capacity. Aerobic exercise practised over a few months, with herbal and dietary support, can quickly improve and strengthen a poor water line. Any activity that requires movement in cooperation with others, like running in a group, dance, and Zumba, not only improve heart and circulation, but also teach trust and social skills. A poor water line can be improved by learning to tune in to ones feelings and to develop non-logical awareness through art, singing in a choir, or developing spiritual awareness within a supportive group.

Sources

American Heart Association. *Is Broken Heart Syndrome Real?* (Dallas, TX: American Heart Association, 13 May 2024). https://www.heart.org/en/health-topics/cardiomyopathy/what-is-cardiomyopathy-in-adults/is-broken-heart-syndrome-real

Cook, J. "The Science That Proves Grief Can Damage Your Body as Well as Your Mind: From Heart Disease to Rheumatoid Arthritis – Evidence Links Bereavement to a Raft of Conditions." *Daily Mail*, 20 March 2023. https://www.dailymail.co.uk/health/article-11882537/The-science-proves-grief-damage-body-mind.html

Daily Mail. "Heartbreak Can Kill You: Grief from Losing a Loved One Causes Deadly Inflammation, Study Reveals." *Dail Mail*, 23 October 2018. https://www.dailymail.co.uk/health/article-6307795/Heartbreak-kill-Grief-losing-loved-one-causes-deadly-inflammation-study-reveals.html

Harvard Health Publishing. "Gum Disease and Heart Disease: The Common Thread." *Heart Health*, 15 February 2021. https://www.health.harvard.edu/heart-health/gum-disease-and-heart-disease-the-common-thread

13

The fire line

The meaning, metaphor, and nature of the fire line

The fire line (Figure 13.1) is called either the fate line, the Saturn line, or sometimes the destiny line in traditional palmistry. It is the most difficult major line to identify, as usually it's fainter than the other major lines and is easily the most variable in length. Often it's broken, scratchy, or partially missing. It is common for it not to appear on the hands until the age of 30 or so. This line strengthens and lengthens as we grow to maturity.

The fire line begins in the lower half of the palm and runs up vertically through the palm's centre towards the middle finger.

Its metaphor is the life path, a track cutting through the forest of life's distractions, forming our individual priorities, values, and aims. It rules character, the sense of who you are, your vocational choices, and what you are dedicated to. Physically it rules the erector spinae (the series of muscles that straighten and rotate the spine). To lack a fire line is to lack backbone, to have no personal goals or values, and not to know what vocation to follow. This line is very varied where it starts. It may begin low down in the centre of the palm, or start somewhere in the middle of the hand, or rise up from the earth line. It is a fully formed line when

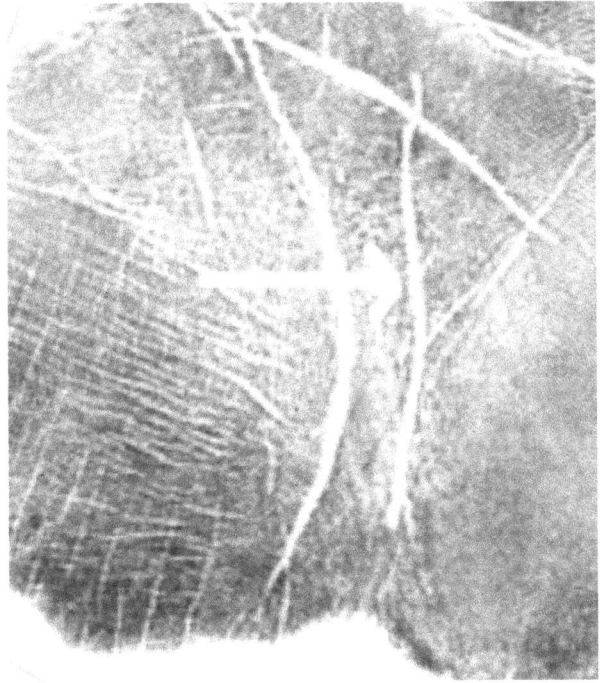

Figure 13.1. The fire line.

it runs from palm base to end on or near the water line. Note that only if the line is pushing up towards the middle finger is it a fire line. Any line running vertically towards other digits is not.

No fire line

Where there is no fire line present (Figure 13.2), this is not a serious issue if the person is under 30 or if this is missing on the passive hand. This means a person is fluid in their character and highly likely to change job, life path, sexuality, or political persuasion – goals and character aren't fixed or certain. The personality isn't strongly defined. They haven't found themselves. Without a

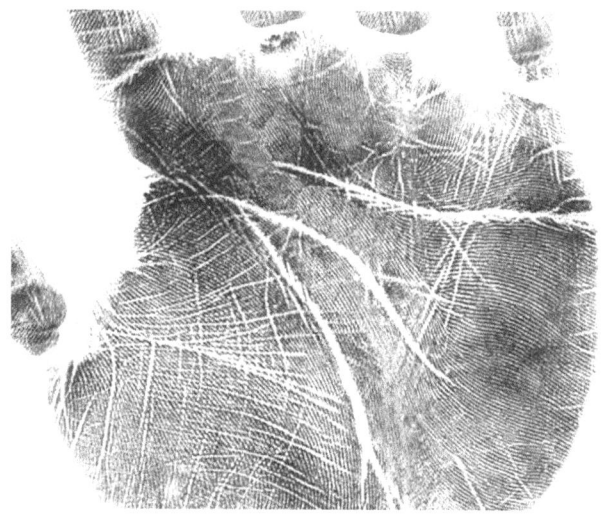

Figure 13.2.   Palm with no fire line.

fire line, one is uncertain of what job, life choices, and path to take in life.

Hands with no fire lines often linger in university until their thirties, then work in team-orientated, structured fields that provide an extension of the school environment, like social work, teaching, or local government. The lack of a fire line means that there is little in the way of personal ethics and beliefs. It is an irony that many who furiously advocate a cause, actually conform to crowd values: devout followers of fashion, cult, or coven usually lack a fire line and don't actually have a personal sense of values at all.

The lack of a fire line is at the heart of much behaviour that is immature and incoherent and is a leading sign of psychological illness. The presence of this line gives a sense of balance and acceptance and of taking up the burden of willing responsibility. Modern society presents a plethora of easy ways to define ourselves through simplistic value systems, fashions, political stances and off-the-shelf culture choices so we struggle to blaze our own pathway through endless possibilities. Prevailing culture is so powerful in its pressures that it overwhelms us. People more than ever lack "backbone", and fire lines are becoming poorer in quality, are developing later and are frequently missing. This of course indicates that spinal problems are endemic. The cost of dealing with back pain in the UK in the past ten years has tripled (Rachel Suff, *Spinal Conditions in the UK*).

Islands in the fire (Figure 13.3) line indicate periods of dissatisfaction and frustration with work or life in general, and often financial difficulties or a sense of losing one's way. The spine is often highlighted as an issue with a large island, particularly in the lumbar vertebrae, if the island is in the lower part of the line. A chained formation (made up of lots of small islands) weakens the line considerably and lessens the ability to support oneself and keep psychologically stable.

Breaks in the line are quite common: curiously, they don't indicate spinal problems, but change in life direction. This often means a new career, and if the second section of the line is angled differently, a very different set of priorities and a different type of vocation. The condition of the line following the break is a guide to how successful this change is.

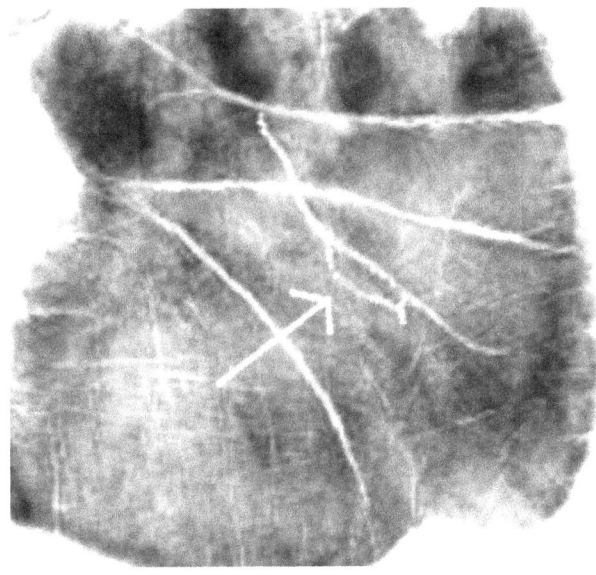

Figure 13.3. Island in the fire line.

Halfway there

It is common to see the fire line only appearing halfway up the palm (Figure 13.4), coinciding with the age of 35 or so (timing is crude on this line but where it crosses the air line is around 40 and where it crosses the water line, around 60). This indicates of a sense of direction and purpose arriving at around this age.

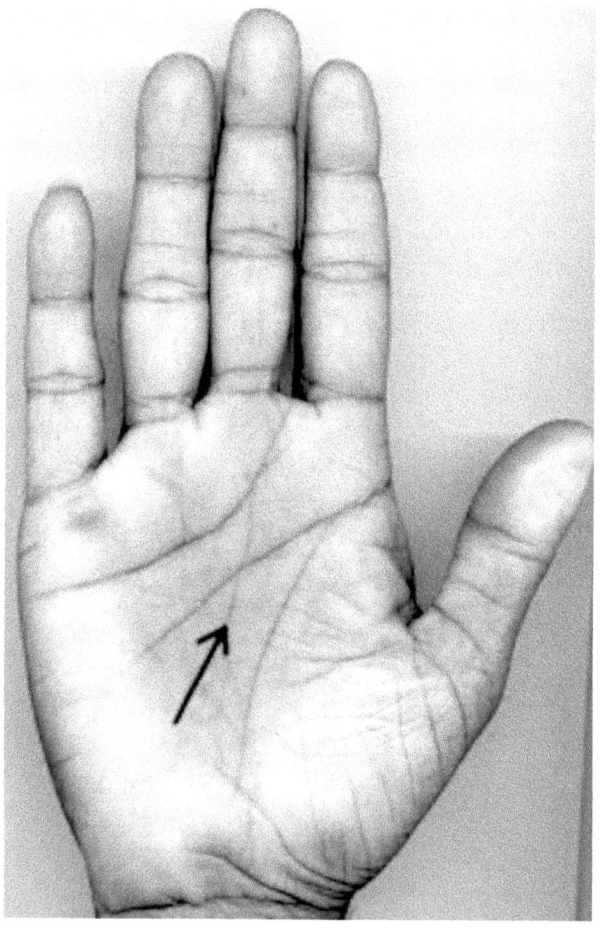

Figure 13.4. Fire line beginning halfway up the hand.

Often those with this pattern will say it wasn't till mid-life that they "found themselves" and knew what they wanted to do with their life.

The fire line can also be present in the bottom half of the hand, but not in the top half, above the air line. On a person under 40 this isn't an issue – the line will probably grow as the person ages. However on a 60-year-old's palm, this would represent a loss of a sense of purpose, ambition, and passion for work in mid-life.

Going all the way – complete crossing fire lines

Very occasionally, you'll find the line running all the way from the base of the palm to the base of the middle digit (Figure 13.5). Like all lines that cross the palm completely, this creates an obsessive pattern, so the bearer feels fixed and bound to the same life path, job, and duty. They become stuck in life patterns, feeling fatalistic and that life presents few options. There is an amazing strength in all crossing major lines, and in this case the ability to keep going, never shirking duty, obligation, and work, is admirable. However, their life can easily become one of routine and duty. The spine tends to seize, and the muscles supporting it become fixed and immobile. The completely crossing line indicates an eventual spinal issue later in life, where the rigidity of the spine causes disc issues. All around will love them for their reliability, sense of duty, and steadfastness, but they themselves may feel trapped. If this pattern is on the passive palm, obligation to family will come before everything.

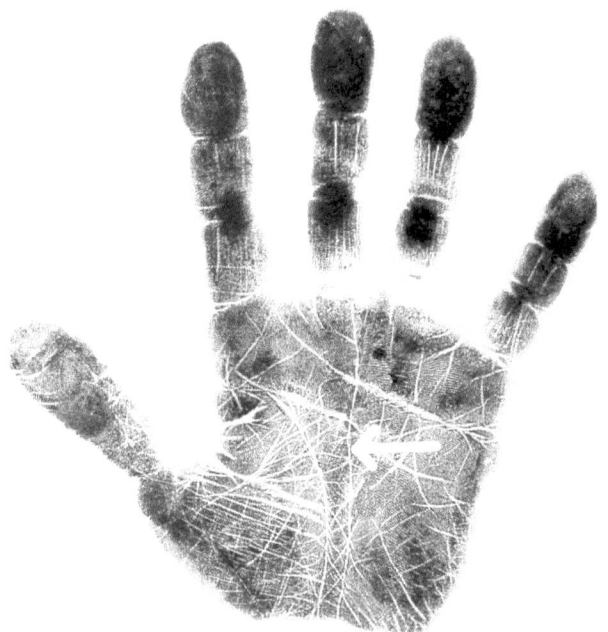

Figure 13.5. Complete crossing fire line: a fire line that crosses the palm completely. This man has fused vertebrae in the lumbar spine and has been a building surveyor for 38 years.

Burning up scratchy, striated fire lines

When you see the fire line made up of a series of little scratches, this is perhaps the most negative sign in health terms (Figure 13.6). This marking is, perhaps unexpectedly, a sign of a super-successful person "burning up" as they plough through life. It is as if the fire line is scorching its way along, blazing out of control, giving a striving, stressful attitude to work and achievement. This is a careerist whose job lends status and prestige; but it's about getting an identity through success, rather than knowing who one is and what one really wants. It is common in those sexy, high-

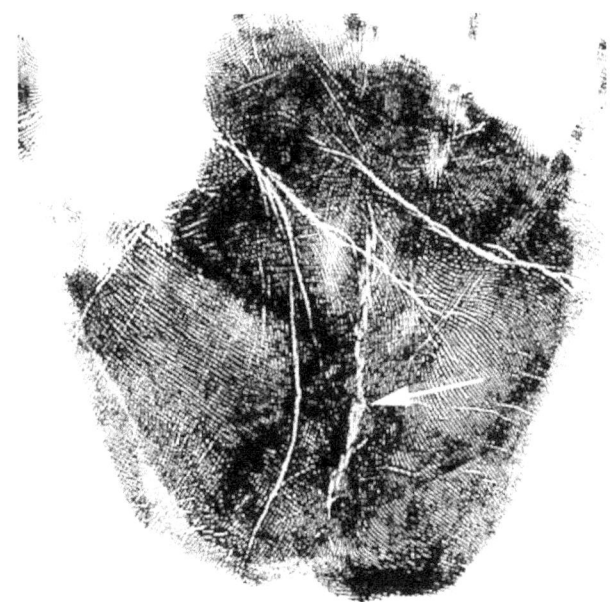

Figure 13.6. Palm of a TV executive who had a breakdown and retired at 51.

profile vocations – the media, finance, TV, law, PR, advertising, web influencers- and so on. Those with striated fire lines are burning with a brilliant light and make fortunes and climb great heights. However, they are extremely liable to break down, burn out, and to get spinal and gut and prolapse issues. Practically everyone I have seen with this sign has eventually suffered some form of physical and mental collapse.

Where the fire line originates from the earth line (Figure 13.7), this shows someone who bases their goals on their "root": their background, family, and education. Such personalities are highly conventional; they often work in the same profession as their parents or the government in some way. It is as if they've internalised a set of values from their formative influences and feel bound to them. Status is conferred upon them from an exterior source, and they march on the road placed before them in life.

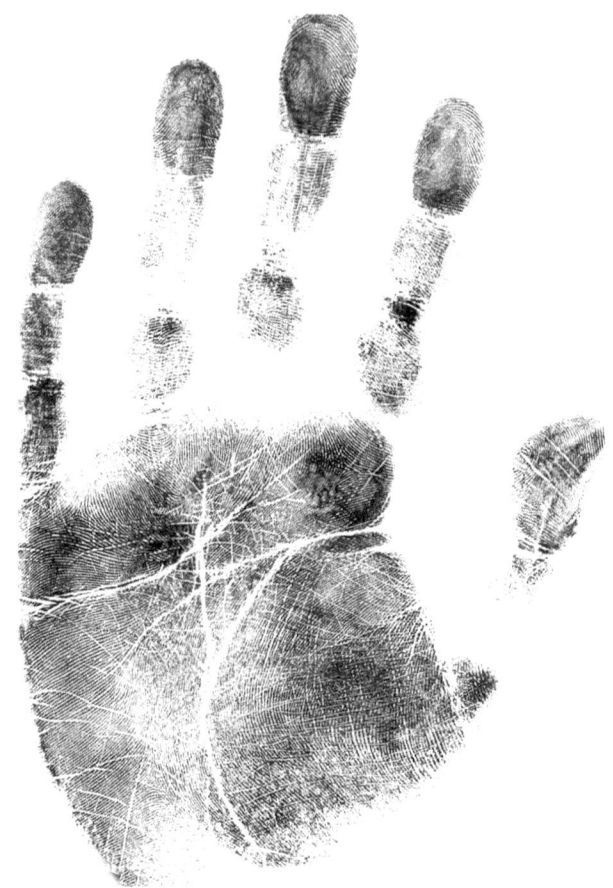

Figure 13.7. Fire line beginning on earth line on a government official.

Fire fills the earth

A difficult development healthwise is where the fire line replaces a section of the earth line (Figure 13.8).

When this pattern occurs, earth line qualities – structure, home, roots, and stability – are secondary to vocation. This means that home, family, and health are all at the mercy of the demands of work. This is someone who will move house, sacrifice their health,

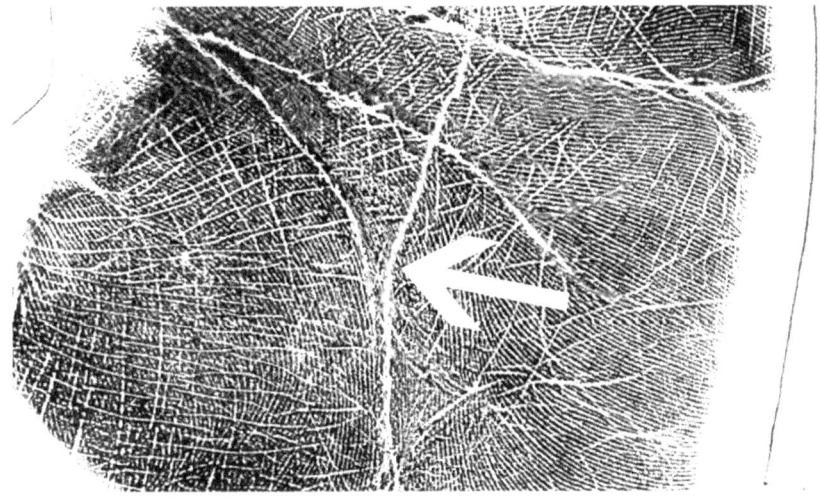

Figure 13.8. Fire line replacing section of earth line.

move heaven and earth for their vocation, because they feel that work *is* life. It is vital to impress upon anyone with this line that they must put health, family, and stability above the demands of work, as health issues will be extremely common in later life. This is a definite warning sign on the active hand of someone literally "working themselves to death". It is very important to impress upon them the need to prioritise their health, and to have regular check-ups. This is one of the clearest signs of eventual health problems in the hand, and from the age of 60 onwards, those with this marking are very commonly beset with serious health problems.

Building a fire line

This line can develop quickly. Always advise those with no fire line to define a personal physical goal – to lose ten kilos, say, or to learn to ski, or learn salsa to a pro level: it must be something difficult but something they can physically progress towards. Then they must work to develop that quality, no matter what distractions, difficulties, and drawbacks beset them. This is how a life path is formed – by forcing a personal goal through the forest of easy opportunity. Also advise people without this line to define themselves by keeping a personal journal: one that records with absolute honesty, not events, but their own insights, reflections, and feelings; in such manner is self-definition realised. Note that if this line's missing, that is not a sign of a lack of success – only that one cannot be successful on one's own terms. The strength of the line indicates how well entrenched you are in your own values, how protected you are from the common, corporate, or received ideals.

Sources

Rachel Suff, *Health Report: Spinal Conditions in the UK* (London: Chartered Institute of Personnel and Development, 23 January 2020).

RCGP. *Research Needed to Explore Reasons for Increase in People Unable to Work Due to Back Pain, Says RCGP*. (London: Royal College of General Practitioners, 19 January 2024). https://www.rcgp.org.uk/News/Research-needed-work-back-pain

14

Minor lines

Major points of the minor lines

Unlike the major lines, which are practically always present in some form, any given palm may have no minor lines at all. A palm with coarse skin and crude major lines will often have none. On any given palm, you'll usually find a lot of minor lines, but again, not all will be present. The minor lines are always half-formed, scratchy, and much fainter than the major ones.

Minor lines change much more quickly than major ones (often within a week or two). They are seams of gold for the medical palmist, as certain lines are crucial health barometers.

Where you find the rare case of a minor line being the *strongest*, *deepest*, *clearest* line on a palm (Figure 14.1) – when it's more marked than any of the major lines – then there is a problem. This will always have a medical manifestation. The person's life force (as represented by the major lines) is overshadowed by an issue that compromises their energetic integrity. They are undermined by a chemical, physical, and psychological imbalance.

If, for example, the allergy line is the strongest line on the palm (this line is discussed later), this would mean a person's whole life experience revolves around diet, health, and allergies.

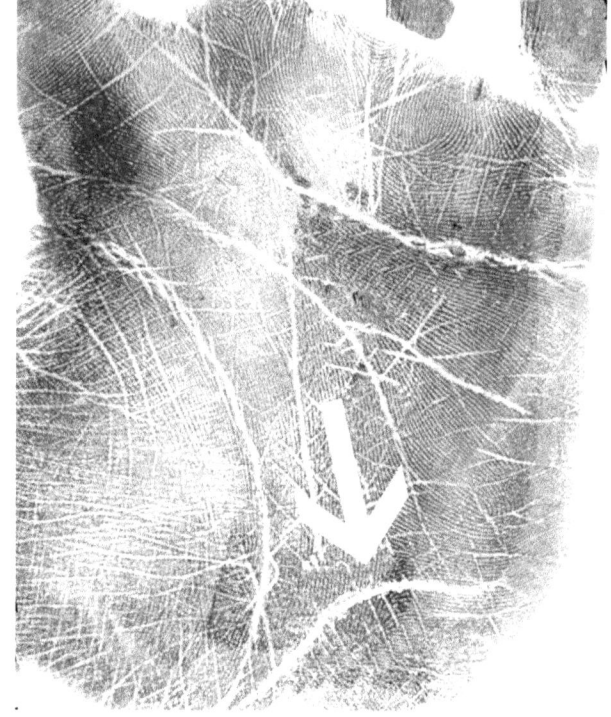

Figure 14.1. A dominant allergy line that is the strongest line on the palm.

It means that they cannot function fully, and that their immune system is hyper-reactive and dominant over everything.

There are ten minor lines that are important in hand-reading practice; however, only certain ones are relevant in health terms. The important lines in medical analysis are the mirage line, the allergy line, the sublimation line, the intensity line; and; in particular, the vagus nerve line. We'll examine them one by one.

Mirage line

The mirage line (Figure 14.2) is traditionally known as the Ring of Saturn, the Girdle of Venus, and, sometimes, the Neptune line. It floats above the water line, and is often fragmentary in form. It is like a second water line of emotional energy, which floats in a surreal air of heightened experience.

The stronger this line is marked, the stronger the drive to escape the mundane to higher realms. The line seeks dreamy experiences, beauty, luxury, perfection, the surreal, and spiritual highs. You could say that this line gives the drive to get "out of your head". There is always a need to attain emotional experiences just out of reach – the most incredible party, the magnificent castle, the exquisite restaurant, the lover who is a mythical, god-like creature. Wherever you see this line, the need to escape reality is strong, and this can mean a love of escapist drug-induced experiences. People with this line strongly marked have usually embarked on at least a few journeys into drug-fuelled hedonism. There is a love of performance, fantasy, dreams, and fancy dress – and places

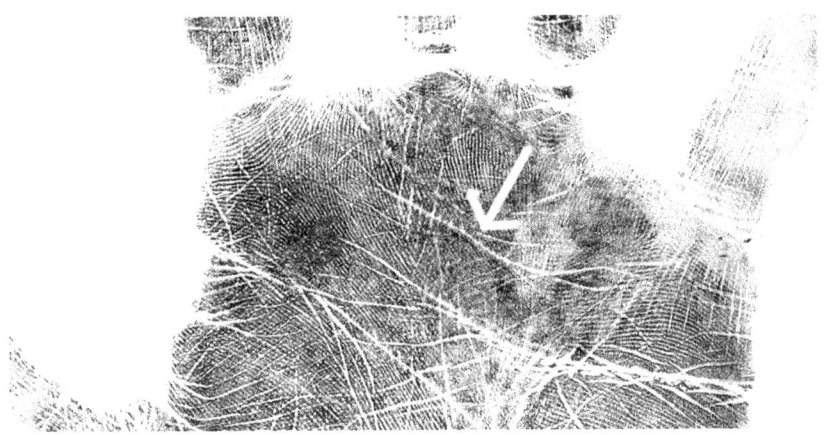

Figure 14.2. A mirage line – often it is more fragmented than it is in this example.

where one can escape the mundane – art galleries, night clubs, online gaming, festivals, fantasy games, escapist films, and literature. Depending on how sensitive and grounded the palm is (check the earth line), this marking can create a decadent escapist or a an inspired creative trying to get to a higher, more perfect place. It is found on those who are fascinated by all things spiritual. There is always a love of myth, magic, astrology, symbols, and visions.

Medically, this line is associated with hypochondria, delusion, psychosis, and a reluctance to face concrete reality. It tends to make a person more inclined towards introversion, to playing out roles of fantasy –those who prefer dreams to reality. It is a sign of a more fragile psychology and is found on those who easily slip into unrealistic expectations or fears of unlikely events – for instance, of tidal waves or earthquakes.

When the line is found in fragmented form (Figure 14.3), it tends to produce a hypersensitive, deeply introverted nature. This is a sign of being highly strung. It is important to avoid loud, chaotic experiences, drug-taking, and complex relationships, as this can disorientate them more easily than most. Migraines are strongly linked to this pattern, as well as hypochondria; there is also a tendency to pursue impossible relationships and fantastic

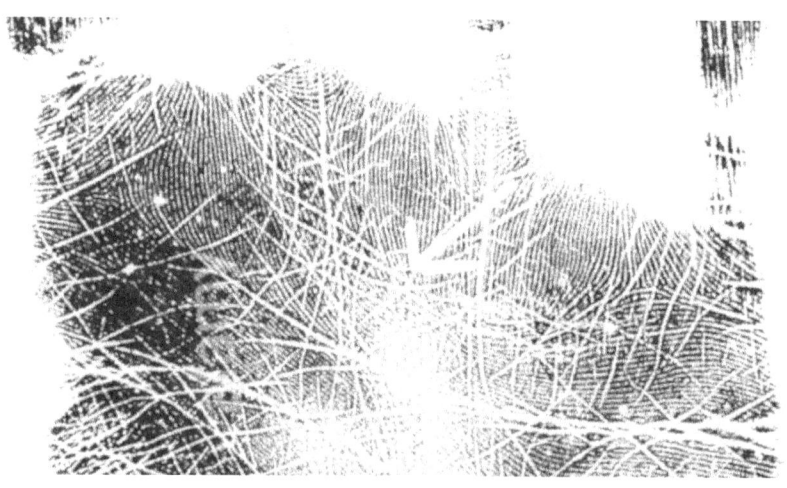

Figure 14.3. Fragmented mirage line.

tinctures, supplements, and miracle cures in order to live more fully. Those with this pattern should try to find a calm, grounded, stable lifestyle and to create a consistent pattern of artistic or spiritual practice, which will clear the fragmented lines before too long.

Vagus nerve line

The vagus nerve line (Figure 14.4) has historically been called the hepatica, the health line, the mercury line, or the liver line, highlighting its significance as an indicator of general health. The line runs vertically up the side of the hand opposite the thumb and moves towards the little finger. Needless to say, this line

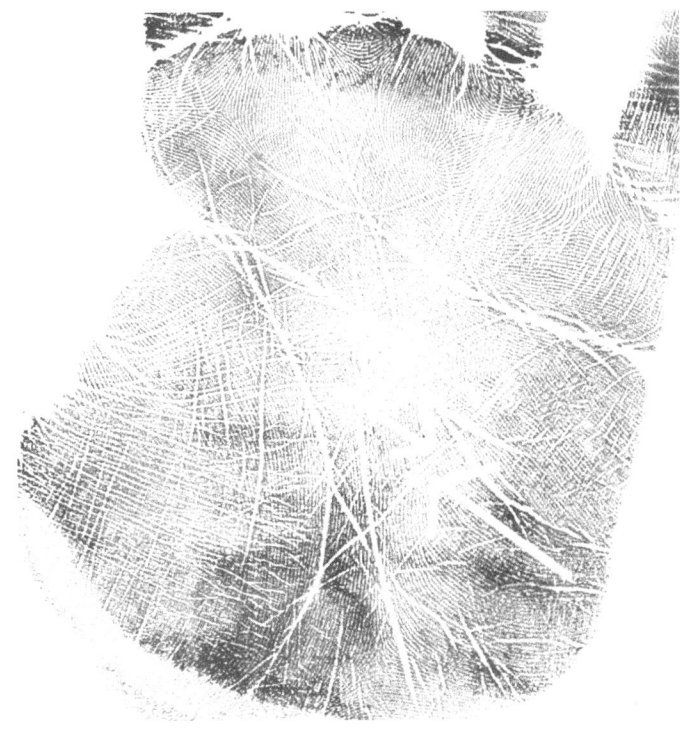

Figure 14.4. The vagus nerve line.

represents the vagus nerve: a major component of the parasympathetic nervous system, which oversees a vast array of crucial bodily functions, including immune response, digestion, and heart rate. It establishes one of the major connections between the brain and the gastrointestinal tract and sends information about the state of the inner organs to the brain.

The line tends to get progressively thicker, scratchier and more broken up as we sink into old age – becoming slowly more dominant (Figure 14.5). Stomach acid decreases by half after 50 years of age and dyspepsia, digestive ills, constipation, and various nervous and inflammatory conditions tend to haunt the elderly. All too often the over-sixties tend to suffer from "nerves", lung problems, poor sleep, and poor digestion. Many an oldie has to think very carefully before having another piece of cake or munching peanuts.

In our frantic, over excitable world, it's not unusual to find this line in fragmented form on the palms of people of all ages. A broken or highly fragmented vagus line is very common and merely shows that the body is not functioning at its optimum.

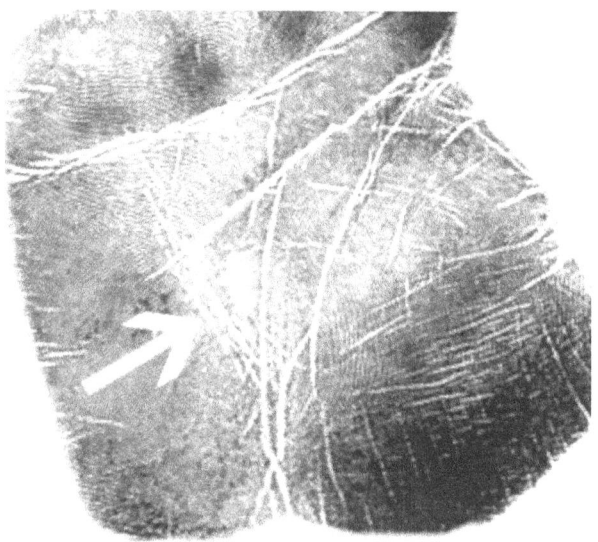

Figure 14.5. Vagus nerve line on a 68 year old.

Most defects in the line will be found to suggest a disorder in the organs of digestion or respiration and internal inflammation.

Islands in this line (Figure 14.6) are a worrying sign, indicating a period when the constitution is running at a low ebb, suggesting a predisposition to chest infections and problems with the respiratory system. A chained line indicates general debility and a weakened constitution.

Very occasionally, you'll see a vagus nerve line that is long, clear, and fine. This is an excellent indicator, healthwise, as it shows someone with a good connection to their deep physical processes. A clear, fine line gives very fine motor and breathing control and the ability to think laterally. There is a fascinating capacity to come up with original and inspired ideas. It is common on inventors, original thinkers, inspired teachers, writers, and yoga and meditation practitioners (Figure 14.7). It is interesting to note that in China, where the elderly often practice tai chi in the open air, the vagus nerve line appears in very fine, clear condition on most participants.

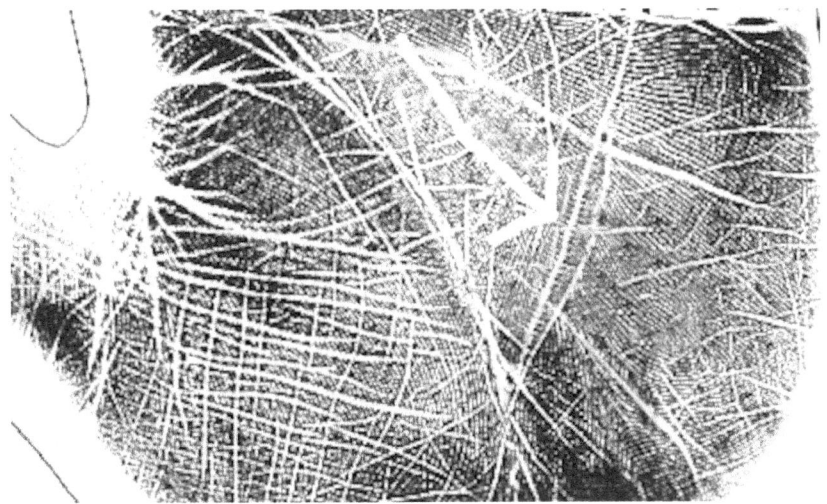

Figure 14.6. Island in the vagus nerve line on a woman who has suffered a series of lung infections.

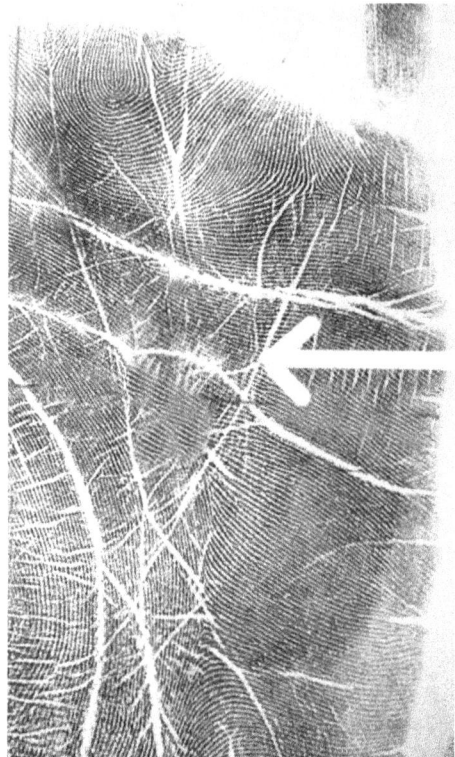

Figure 14.7. A yoga practitioner's vagus nerve line.

The vagus nerve line can be improved very quickly. Attention to digestion is essential – making sure the stomach is never over-full or over-acidic, with attention given to what can be properly digested and assimilated. Also, controlling the breath through deep breathing exercises and calming techniques will make a huge difference. (See Figures 14.8 and 14.9.)

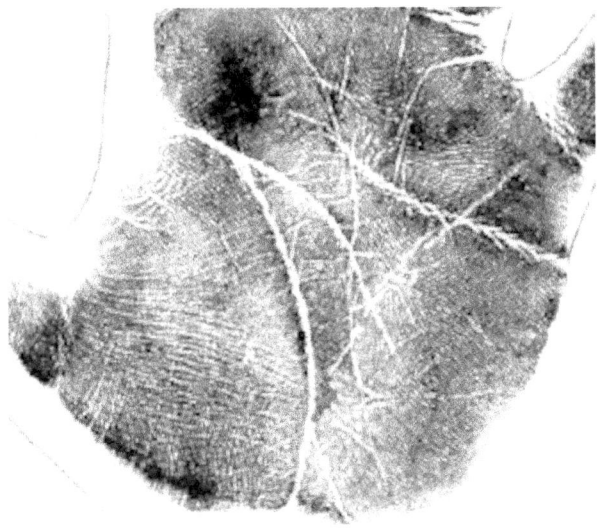

Figure 14.8. Vagus nerve line before kundalini meditation course.

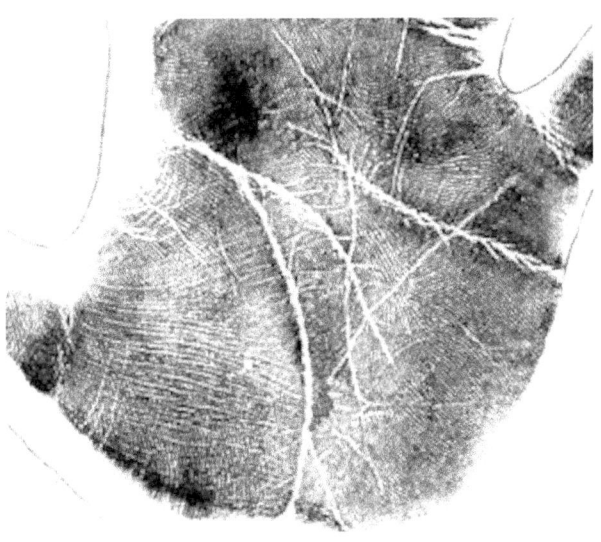

Figure 14.9. Vagus line after seven months of daily practice.

Sublimation line

This line is called the Apollo line or line of sun in traditional palmistry. It was thought to show fame and public adoration. In fact, it is a reflection of the depth of someone's capacity to sublimate themselves in an activity. It is a sign of being able to forget oneself, inner harmony and a sense of stillness. This is always found through a practice, skill or hobby, or simply just being, still and alone in perfect peace.

The sublimation line (Figure 14.10) is very commonly seen above the water line: as such, it is of no consequence. Only when the line appears *below* the water line for at least two centimetres is it worthy of comment.

When you see this line long and clear, it signifies someone who is content, who has found a way of losing themselves in an activity that gives them a sense of "self-forgetting". It is a wonderfully healing sign to see – often found on those who immerse themselves in an art, hobby, craft, or practice, being "in the moment". It is common on healers, yogis, artists, singers, actors, physical therapists, tai-chi practitioners, or those who lose themselves watching tropical fish for hours on end. It might be seen as a sign of contentment and is an excellent sign (Figure 14.11).

The sublimation line relates to kidney function. In Traditional

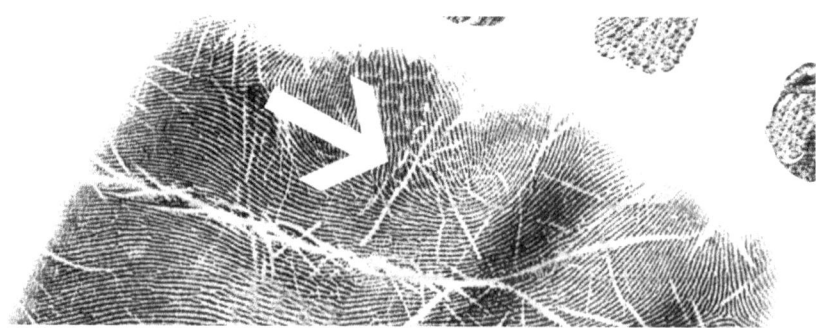

Figure 14.10. Typical sublimation line – this is normal and of no consequence.

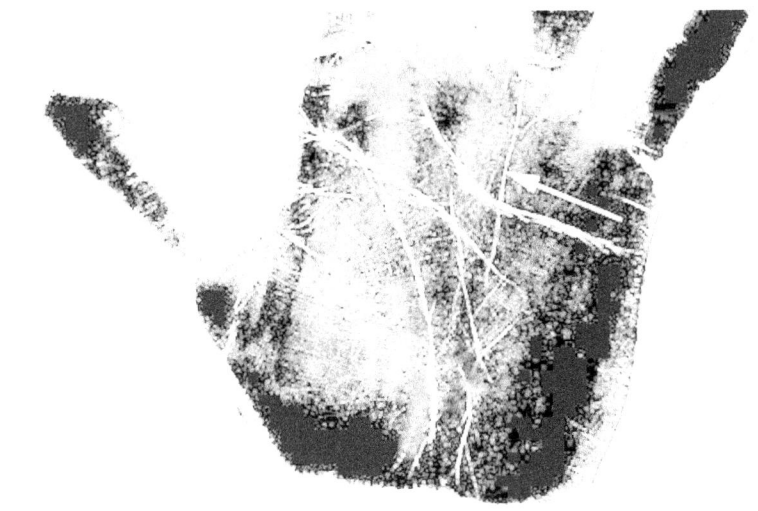

Figure 14.11. Sublimation line on a shiatsu practitioner's hand.

Chinese Medicine the kidneys are vital in that they store and control "essence" and respond negatively to fear. When this line is seen strong and clear it tends to show an absence of fear, a feeling of fulfilment and contentment and is a strong indicator of lack of stress and good kidney health.

Whenever this line is found in clear form, it's a sign that it is essential for this person to regularly withdraw from people into a private space, where they can find a sense of peace.

Intensity line

This line is quite common. It is a thin, straight, horizontal line in the lower area of the hand opposite the Venus mount. It cuts off the deeper, reflective zone of the mind and makes it difficult to relax. People with this line need to seek excitement and movement in order to switch off. It is a sign of high energy and

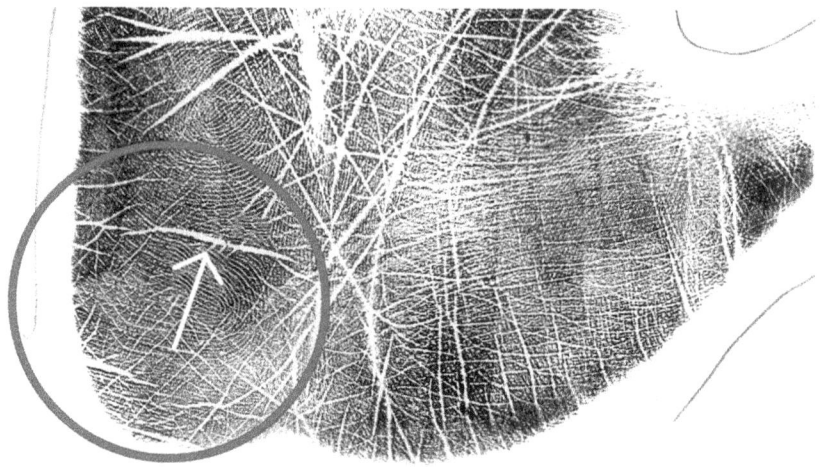

Figure 14.12. Intensity line on a motorcycle racer.

often an obsession with exercise. You'll find this line in parachutists, aerobics instructors, demented dancers, motorcyclists, racing drivers and skiers (Figure 14.12) – they need to do something to stimulate the senses. There is a deep disconnect in the subconscious that means only through physical exhaustion can they truly relax. Often it's a sign of over-active adrenal glands. A programme of calming herbs, acupuncture, and therapy seems to eliminate this marking in time.

Allergy line

Often known as the via lascivia, this line (Figure 14.13) is found in the same place as the intensity line, but it is curved instead of straight and more often than not in a broken-up formation. Sometimes it can run all the way to the earth line, where it's particularly powerful in effect. It indicates a hyper-responsive immune system. The presence of allergies is highly likely, the most common

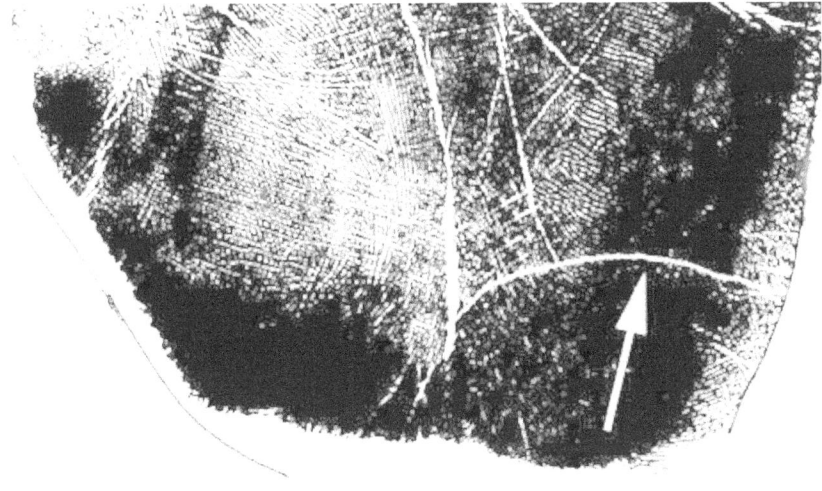

Figure 14.13. An allergy line.

allergens being eggs, wheat, dairy, nuts, and shellfish. There can also be irrational fears, of, for instance, spiders or of deep water. This is a particularly worrying sign if the line is very strong and if there are any signs of weakness of the earth line. This is a marker for all kinds of dietary issues. Whenever this line is seen, it's advisable that the client try some form of elimination diet, so likely allergic reactions are noted when things like dairy or nuts are introduced. It is vital for anyone with this sign to understand what their particular sensitivities are, as it can be a lifelong issue until understood and dealt with.

Random markings

Part of the ancient baggage of palmistry means that people will constantly badger you to interpret a cross or star formation somewhere on their palm, terrified it foretells some dark and dismal outcome. Meanwhile their enormous allergy line, the cause of all their issues, is completely ignored!

Do re-assure anyone who asks that these markings are mostly meaningless. Everyone has the odd squiggle, square, star, or cross somewhere on their palm, it's impossible to categorise them all. Faint marks, triangles, crosses, and so on come and go very quickly. They fact that they may have – for example – a completely crossing water line is massively more important!

As a medical hand analyst, my opinion is that these signs are not relevant, so don't lose your way with random markings: focus on the major health issues found elsewhere.

15

Stress!

The roots of so many health issues lie in high stress levels. A stressed nervous system is like a taut bowstring: in a constant state of alertness and sensitivity to any external stimulus. Such a state is excellent for a momentary situation, such as tackling a charging bear; however, as a permanent condition, such a state is extremely costly, comparable to taking a bazooka to tackle a mosquito. Experienced hand readers find, time and time again, that hands that display high stress levels eventually manifest medical problems. To take just one area of the body, the gut – the gut lends the brain a large amount of energy in order to deal with stress and effectively shuts down when it perceives an emergency, so perennial levels of tension causes stomach cramps, nausea, irritable bowel, and a host of gut problems.

Long-term stress seems to trigger a range of conditions, ranging from hypertension, heart disease, and some types of cancer, to Type II diabetes and arthritis. Even memory loss is associated with stress. The brain's hippocampus (which stores our memories and links them to each other) is densely populated with sensors for stress hormones. If the hippocampus registers high levels of such hormones, the brain cuts the memory facility. After all, if you are running from a predator, you don't need to waste energy remembering which plants you pass by. During stressful times, we develop a kind of tunnel vision—to enable us to direct our attention to the problem at hand. However, in the long term this has a corrosive effect on brain function and the body/mind process.

Stress markers in the hands

The hand is excellent at registering stress levels, and there are many markers that allow us to see how serious is the strain it is putting on a person. Initial observations, like noting a person has an air palm, or silky skin, a tented arch print, or a short air line will alert you to those who have a predisposition to suffer from nervous tension.

The most obvious marker for stress is simply a hand covered in lots of fine lines, combined with rigid fingers that won't bend back. This is particularly important if the lines suddenly become more numerous over a short period of time. When someone's palm has a blizzard of random lines all over (not as part of the major/minor line patterns), then that person must be considered highly anxious and over-stimulated. Try to see lots of lines as flashes of thought, flickers of nervous energy, and surges of adrenalin and cortisone, which drain and confuse the most basic human interaction. Figure 15.1 illustrates how a difficult life situation registers in the hand.

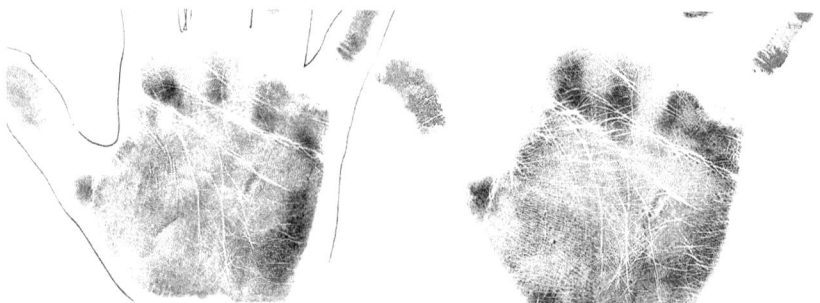

Figure 15.1. Hands of woman before and during a difficult divorce and house move.

You may find one particular area of the palm has more stress lines than the rest of the hand, and this gives a clue to the area of life causing the problems.

If there are loads of crossing stress lines within the semicircle of the earth line on the Venus mount (Figure 15.2), it shows stress and disturbance arising within the home and family environment. These are not particularly important if there are only three or four, as most of us have some of these; but if there are very many, it's a sure sign of domestic stress and family issues, and depletion of minerals and physical resources, leaving a person highly vulnerable to infection and illness.

If the stress lines are running over the area opposite the Venus mount on the lower half of the hand (Figure 15.3), it shows disturbance in the person's inner life – they have fears and issues in expressing and connecting to who they truly are and what they want. Yearned-for children, artistic desires, hidden fears, and unexpressed needs are all locked up here.

A mess of lines under the ring and little finger in the upper half of the hand shows stress about interacting, creativity, performing, communicating, and impressing people, or it could

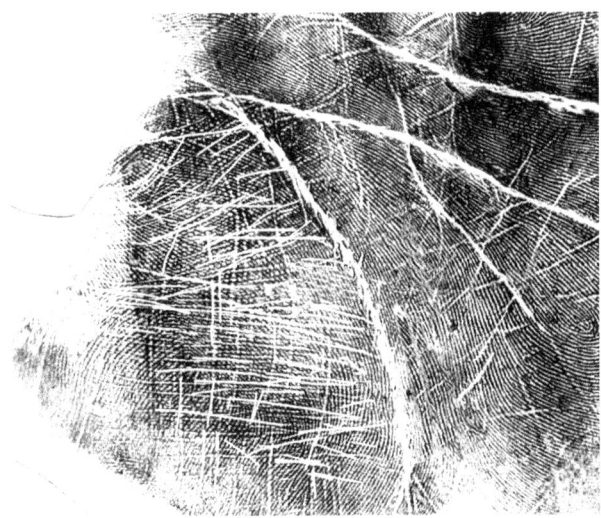

Figure 15.2. Stress lines within the Venus mount.

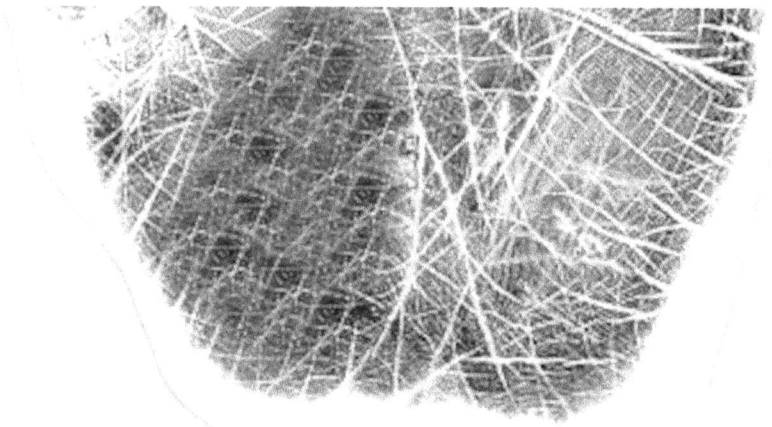

Figure 15.3. Stress lines in the lower quadrant opposite Venus mount.

be about love, intimacy, and sexual issues if nearer the base of the little digit.

If the stress lines are all over the zone beneath the index finger, the conflict is about ambition, ego, and personal values.

Stress markings on the major lines

The air line and the earth line are the most important major lines for indicating stress.

As the air line shows how we think, perceive, and process information, the type and quality of this line can reveal potential strains and mental tension. Having a second air line (Figure 15.4) – though very rare – will always show increased chances of mental overload. An additional air line indicates an ability to think in a second, different way. Although this can be useful, it points towards a mind that is prone to massive levels of overthinking, can give the person excess mental chatter, and may argue with itself, as the two lines give different perspectives. It can double someone's

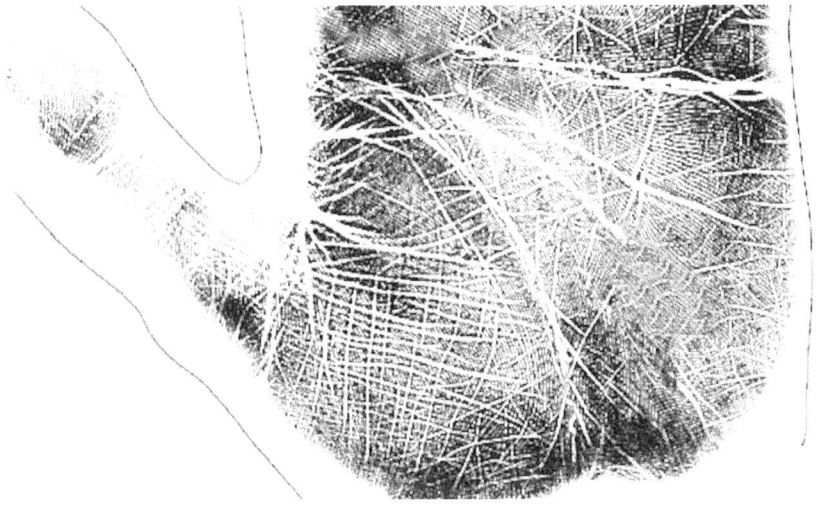

Figure 15.4. Double air lines.

thinking power, but also double someone's capacity to overstress themselves mentally; it is commonly seen on those who have at some time not been able to cope with life issues.

Any deep, plunging air lines that curve steeply down, fragile air lines with fractures, islands, and a broken up quality (Figure 15.5) are all signs of mental sensitivity and someone easily overwhelmed into incoherent mind states.

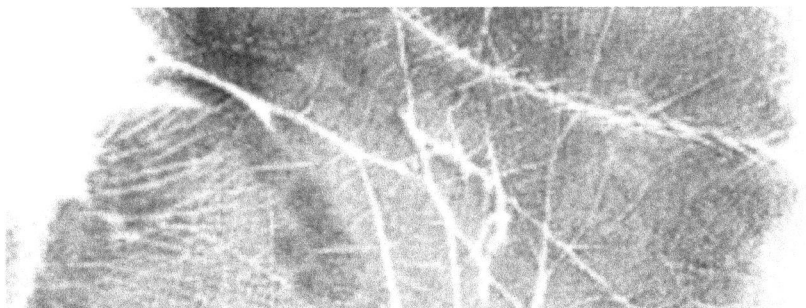

Figure 15.5. Island on the air line of person who has suffered a mental breakdown.

Earth line

The earth line reveals how well we can hold up in terms of stressful situations. If the earth line is weak, high stress indications on any part of the hand indicates, that the gut, stomach and digestion are going to give issues like bloating or diarrhoea. In many ways, the earth line's condition, if strong and clear will indicate that someone can bear stress and keep going, where a weak line will find it much harder to resist physical collapse.

Fire line

As mentioned in Chapter 13, a fractured fire line made up of lots of scratchy lines is a sure sign of eventual burnout.

Minor lines

Any minor lines that are super strong and more marked than all the other lines are a sure sign of stress, imbalance, and the body veering out of kilter. This is particularly true of the vagus nerve line, the intensity line, and the mirage line.

Endocrine system

Although stress can be assessed in lots of areas, one of the most crucial points to examine is the fingertips. Very often there are a few bars and vertical scratch lines on the tips of the fingers, and a some vertical lines on the phalanges – this is normal. However, if the fingertips have a host of these lines, this is important health-wise. The endocrine system is represented by the fingertips: various glands, like the thyroid, thymus, and so on, are indicated here, so a lot of markings show a disturbance in this area. When adolescents enter puberty and when women go through the menopause, the endocrine system goes into overdrive, so it's perfectly normal to see a tempest of markings on the fingertips at such times (see Figure 15.6). However, if neither of these life stages is involved, a high degree of stress and the consequent chemical and imbalance will be creating endocrine problems.

There is some dispute about which finger is related to which specific gland, but the majority of medical hand readers concur that the little finger is associated with the thyroid gland, the ring finger with the thymus, the middle (the longest finger) the pineal, and the index with the pituitary gland.

Figure 15.6. Fingertip markings on a woman going through the menopause.

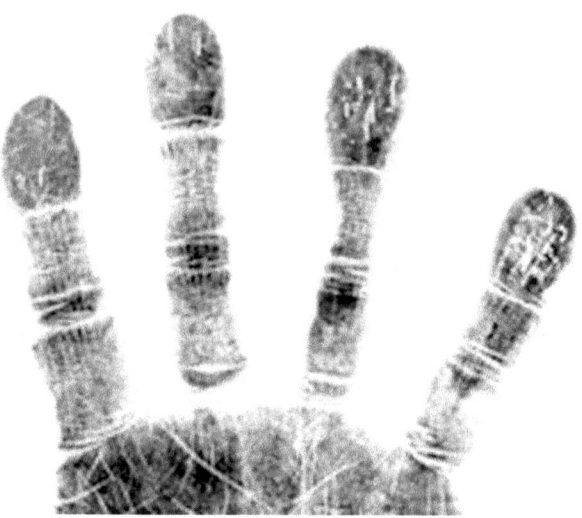

Figure 15.7. Image of the hand of a woman with myasthenia gravis (a disorder of the thymus gland).

As one ages, little lines appear on the fingertips as our systems slow down. However any serious markings on these phalanges *outside puberty or menopause* must be looked at in association with a problem with the respective gland or the endocrine system (Figure 15.7).

Strategies to reduce stress

Stress is probably the most common issue in industrialised nations. According to the UK Mental Health Foundation, over 80% of adults complain of anxiety at some point in their lives.

They recommend certain fundamental steps:

> ▷ *Realize when it is causing you a problem.* You need to make the connection between feeling tired or ill, with the pressures you are faced with. Don't ignore physical warnings such as

tense muscles, over-tiredness, inability to sleep, headaches or migraines.
- *Identify the causes.* Try to identify the underlying causes. Group the possible reasons for your stress into those with a practical solution, those that will get better anyway given time, and those you cannot do anything about. Try to let go of those in the second and third groups – there is no point in worrying about things you cannot change or things that will sort themselves out.
- *Review your lifestyle.* Are you taking on too much? Is someone in your life making things difficult? Are there things you are doing that could be handed over to someone else? Can you do things in a more leisurely way? You may need to prioritise things you are trying to achieve and reorganise your life so that you are not trying to do everything at once.
- *Eat healthily.* There is a growing amount of evidence showing how food affects our mood. Foods to reduce stress include:
  - *bananas* – rich in tryptophan, an amino acid that boosts the formation of serotonin (feel-good hormone) and melatonin (sleep hormone);
  - *spinach* and *broccoli* – replenish magnesium, which lowers stress, as well as Vitamins B and folic acid, which reduces anxiety, panic, and depression;
  - *milk* and *yogurt* – high in calcium, Vitamin B, which is essential for the health of nerves, and tryptophan;
  - a glass of warm *milk* before going to bed – assists with sleep;
  - *tuna* and *mackerel* – rich in omega-3 fatty acids, which control adrenalin and protect the heart;
  - *blueberries* – rich in antioxidants and vitamin C which are stress relievers.
- *Avoid sugar-rich and fatty foods* like ice cream, which leach minerals and affect blood sugar and mood.
- *Cut down smoking and drinking.* Even though they may seem to reduce tension, this is misleading, as they often make problems worse.

- *Exercise.* Proven to be very effective in relieving stress. Even going out to get some fresh air and doing some light physical exercise, like walking to the shops, can help.
- *Take time out.* Take time to relax. Saying "I just can't take the time off" is of no use if you are forced to take time off later through ill health. Striking a balance between responsibility to others and responsibility to yourself is important in reducing stress levels.
- *Be mindful.* Mindful meditation can be practised anywhere at any time. Research has suggested that it can reduce the effects of stress, anxiety, and other related problems, such as insomnia, poor concentration, and low moods. The "Be Mindful" website features a free, specially-developed online course in mindfulness, as well as details of local courses in your area (https://www.nhs.uk/mental-health/self-help/tips-and-support/mindfulness/).
- *Get restful sleep.* Sleeping issues are common when you are suffering from stress. For tips on getting a good night's sleep, read the online guide "How to Sleep Better" (https://www.nhsinform.scot/mind-to-mind/sleeping-better/how-to-sleep-better/)
- *Don't be too hard on yourself.* Try to keep things in perspective. After all, we all have bad days.

16

Skin ridge break-up, string of pearls

The great hand-reading pioneer, Noel Jaquin, discovered an early health warning system by observing the breaking up of the skin ridges that cover the inner palm and also form the fingerprints (Figure 16.1). He found this to be an early sign of bacterial infection or pre-existing condition and called this the "string-of-pearls" effect. Various studies and other hand readers, including Eugene Scheimann – a qualified doctor – have endorsed Jaquin's findings.

Digestive problems, cancer, infections, conditions in the rheumatic family, and many other problems manifest in a disin-

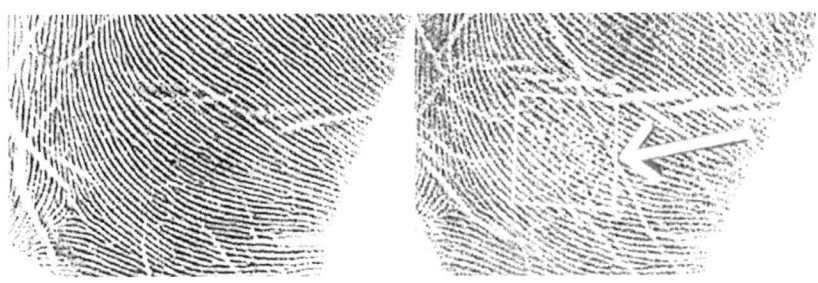

Figure 16.1. Normal and broken-up skin ridges.

tegration of the ridges of the inner palm skin a long time before any physical manifestation. Skin disintegration shows circuits of the nervous system no longer functioning at an optimum level. Jaquin states that faults of the endocrine system may be the cause, as he contends that a perfect glandular system does not, for instance, allow cancer. The failure may be due to high levels of stress in the autonomic nervous system, or some form of poisoning by bacteria, poor diet, or mineral imbalance. The pattern of broken ridges is only visible with a magnifying glass, and you need to make sure to take clear ink handprints of good quality without smudges or missing patches.

Through the magnifying glass, healthy skin looks like a series of raised clean lines of dermal ridges. In certain areas these ridges may be eroded and broken up. They look, when magnified, like a series of dots. There may be fine "veiling" (which is a plethora of very fine lines), so that skin ridges may have the appearance of being erased away. This creates dermal lines that are non-continuous, with a broken up, smudged look.

Dermal ridge erosion

When you discover an area of dermal ridge erosion, always make sure that no outside effect, such as a sporting activity or manual work has caused this effect. Those who use a walking stick for instance, will often develop a band of thick, worn skin ridges in the centre of the palm where they push onto the stick. It is always worth checking that there isn't some hobby or craft that has created broken skin ridges through repetition of particular hand movement.

The area of the palm where the broken ridges occurs signifies cellular damage or less than optimum conditions in the organs corresponding with the section of the hand related to that organ or part of the body. There is not complete agreement among the

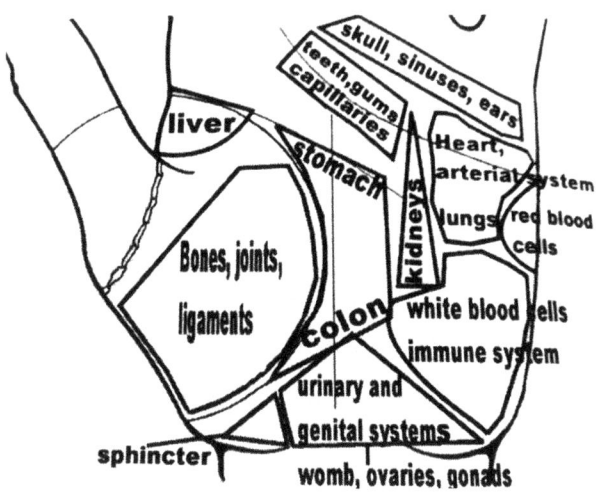

Figure 16.2. Map of the palm and corresponding organs.

various studies and palm readers about exactly which part of the hand relates to which bodily function. All studies however agree that the lower part of the palm relates to the lower parts of the body – the base of the spine, oculogenital area and rectum and the higher area beneath the fingers relates to the upper body, chest and heart area. All confirm the zone around the earth line corresponds to the gut, and that the lower part of the palm opposite the Venus mount relates to the immune system.

Figure 16.2 gives the most consistent correspondences between the organs and areas of the hand from a physiological perspective.

This is remarkably similar to the areas of the body mapped in the palms in hand reflexology (Figure 16.3), although again, there are various different charts available from different schools, systems, and books of reflexology.

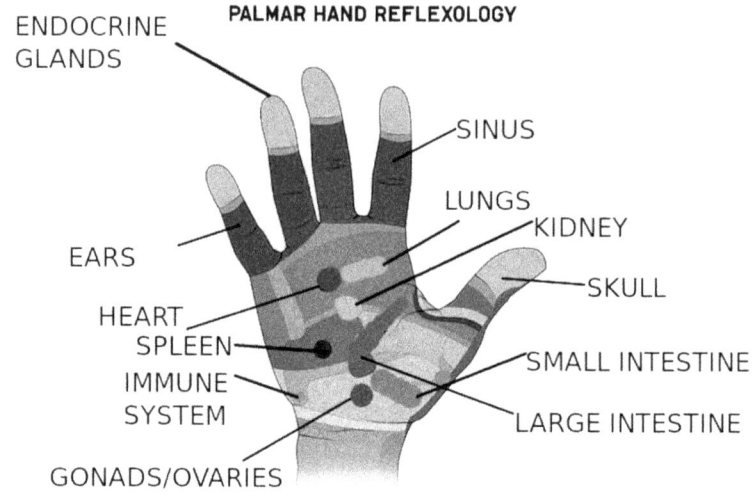

Figure 16.3. Hand reflexology chart.

The "string of pearls"

The "string of pearls" effect is most often seen in the area close to the earth line (Figure 16.4). Research dating back to the early 1970s by various palm readers shows a particular correlation between the appearance of broken ridges around the earth line and the incidence of coeliac disease. Typically, the number of broken-up lines increases with age as gut integrity continues to deteriorate. Fascinating, though, is that in many cases, these white lines begin to vanish with the maintenance of a gluten-free diet. Some researchers believe that white lines are a useful indicator of a person's response to diet therapy, although complete improvement of the print ridges might take as long as two years.

Whenever lots of skin ridge deterioration occurs around the earth line area it's a good idea to advise the patient to meet with a naturopathic physician to investigate digestive health. The best and most appropriate individual diet can make a world of difference in correcting digestive problems, restoring gut integrity, and rebalancing stomach and intestinal bacteria.

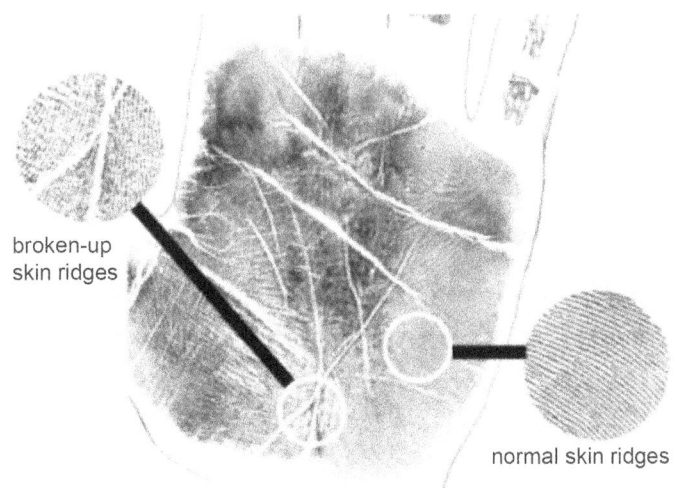

Figure 16.4. Skin ridge break-up around the earth line.

Where there is a serious medical intervention on a particular organ there can be no doubt about the implications of the dermal ridges indicating corresponding organic issues (Figure 16.5).

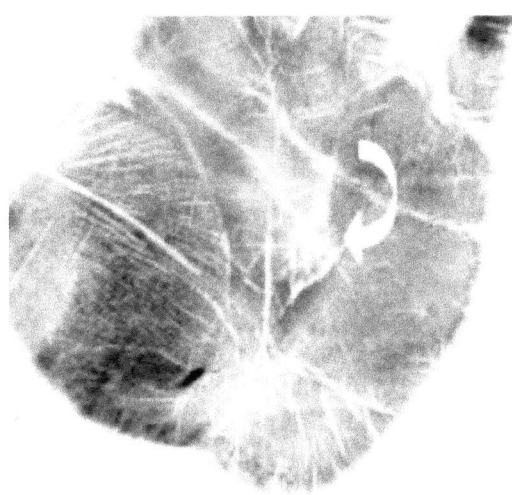

Figure 16.5. The hand of a 46-year-old male who had a kidney transplant three weeks prior to the print being taken.

17

Involuntary hand tremors

We can now move to signals of active disease processes. The medical issues suspected in earlier chapters can be verified in this and Chapter 18, on the fingernails.

Doctors are trained in identifying various conditions indicated by various types of small hand movements. These involuntary quivering patterns of the hand — known as tremors — can be symptoms of various types of nervous disorders, brain diseases, and certain toxic states. There are four basic varieties of tremor. We will examine each one in turn.

Parkinson's tremor

This is easily recognised from the so-called "pill-rolling" movement of the index finger and the thumb (as if holding a pill and rolling it around continuously). The trembling is coarse and of large amplitude, there are usually 4–8 movements a second. This tremor is present while the person is at rest, and it's increased by excitement. Occasionally it stops when the patient uses their hands. It is the most characteristic symptom of Parkinson's. Other signs include: tiny handwriting; a diminished sense of smell; difficulty in sleeping; trouble walking or moving; and a very soft or low voice.

Cerebellar tremor

This is really a twitch that is fine and rhythmic. It is completely absent at rest and becomes evident when the person attempts a deliberate and precise movement, such as putting toothpaste on a brush or lifting a cup to their mouth. It is often called intention tremor. It is an important diagnostic sign of the possibility of multiple sclerosis.

Toxic tremor

This type occurs in poisoning or intoxication from various sources, such alcohol, barbiturates, various chemicals, pesticides, and narcotics. It is a series of shudders and minor tremors that extends to the arms as well as the hands. It appears around 8–12 hours after exposure and disappears slowly as the toxin leaves the system.

Liver tremor

This is a symptom of serious liver issues. It resembles the Parkinson tremor except it's not associated with any type of bodily rigidity or difficulty in movement (very characteristic of Parkinson disease). A major defining feature of this type is that it is increased greatly when the patient holds their arms out at their sides when it becomes exaggerated and resembles a wing-beating motion.

Thyroid tremor

A sign of an overactive thyroid gland is fine trembling that is greatly amplified if the individual stretches and spreads their fingers. The hand is characteristically always wet and warm and has ultra-smooth, satin-like skin.

Nervous tremor

Nervous tremor is the most common form of tremor. This trembling of the fingers is associated with fear, anxiety, and hysteria. Unlike the others, this tremor has no pattern. It is not rhythmical but coarse and irregular and often manifests as a series of shudders that run up the arms. To differentiate this tremor from another, the subject would be given a tranquilliser and their reaction monitored. If the trembling stops, this is almost certainly a nervous tremor.

Sources

AlMuammar, S. A., Noorsaeed, A. S., Alafif, R. A., et al. "The use of internet and social media for health information and its consequences among the population in Saudi Arabia." *Cureus*, Vol. 13, No. 9 (2021): e18338.

Deusch, G., Bain, P., & Brin, M. "Consensus statement of the Movement Disorder Society on tremor. Ad hoc Scientific Committee. *Movement Disorders,* Vol. 13 (1998): 2–23.

Eysenbach, G., & Kohler, C. "What is the prevalence of health-related searches on the World Wide Web? Qualitative and quantitative analysis of search engine queries on the Internet." *AMIA Annual Symposium Proceedings* (February 2003): 225–229.

Rajput, A. H., & Rajput, A. "Medical treatment of essential tremor." Journal of Central Nervous System Disease, Vol. 6 (2014): 29–39.

Smaga, S. "Tremor." *American Family Physician*, Vol. 68, No. 8 (2003): 1545–5552.

18

The nails

The significance of nails as indicators of health status was recognised as early as the fifth century B.C. Nails are often referred to as the barometer of overall health and are an essential aspect of medical hand diagnosis. The manufacture of the nail is an ongoing process, each nail taking roughly six months to grow from cuticle to top edge. It is because the nails are continually being made that they respond so instantly to any hiccups in their growth process (interruptions to the blood supply, poor diet, a sudden shock that rocks the nervous system), registering either in the fabric of the nail or in the pigmentation of the bed beneath.

The fingernails are made of a protein called keratin, found throughout the animal kingdom as hair, claws, feathers, hooves, and horns. The function of the nail is primarily a protective one, guarding the nerve-rich, sensitive tip of the finger against injury. When we are young, our nails grow faster than when we are old. In the summer they put on a greater spurt than they do in the winter. Right-handers will find that they have to file down the nails on their right hands more frequently than those on their left (and vice versa for left-handers). The thumbnails grow the fastest and the little finger's nails the slowest.

- The *nail bed* is part of the nail matrix and lies beneath the nail – It contains blood vessels, nerves, and melanin-producing cells.

> The *nail plate* is the hard shell of the nail itself.
> The *cuticle* is the ridge of skin around the base of the fingernail, situated between the skin of the finger and the nail plate, fusing these structures together and providing a waterproof barrier.

The nail's moons are known as lanula – the white semicircle at the base of the nail. This half-moon appearance is due to the nail bed being tightly packed with keratin (Figure 18.1).

Nails should be examined under natural light and without any protective coating, such as nail polish or nail extensions. Any serious issue will be present on *all* the nails: any pattern or discolouration on a single nail should be ignored. The colour of fingernails should be a healthy rose-pink colour with a soft sheen and a pliable but strong consistency. The moons should be partially visible on most digits. Nails in such condition represent a snapshot of a person's good health over the previous six months,

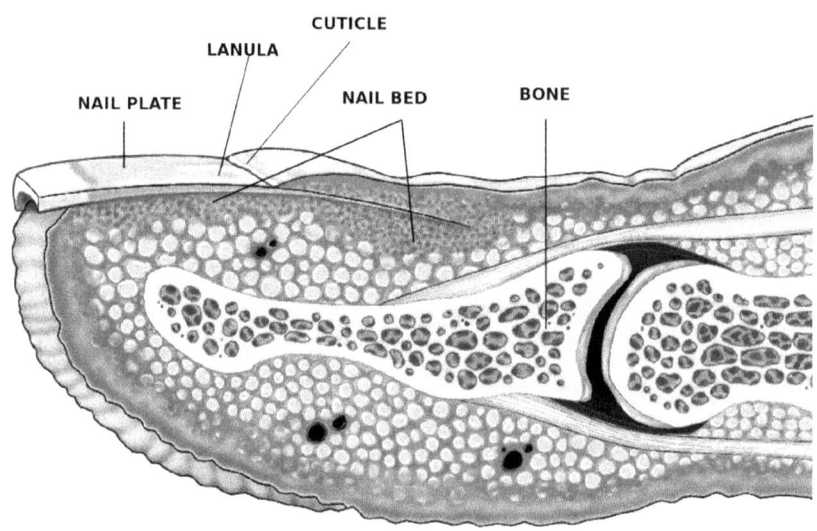

Figure 18.1. The fingernail cross section.

Quick underlying health check using the nails

This test is used in clinical practice and is known as the capillary nail refill test, sometimes known as blanching. This is a quick way of checking circulation and blood supply issues. Press your thumb firmly onto the nail bed just above the moon. Pressure is applied until the nail turns white and the outline of the moon vanishes. This indicates that the blood has been forced from the tissue. Once the tissue has blanched, pressure is removed. The practitioner measures the time it takes for blood (and colour) to return to the tissue; the finger should return to its pink shade in around 2 seconds or less. Blanch time that is much greater than 2 seconds may indicate dehydration, shock, early peripheral vascular disease, or hypothermia.

Alarming fungal infections

Onychomycosis

Some of the most alarming looking conditions, where the fingernails are deeply discoloured and appear corroded, crumbling or flaking apart are actually the least serious, as these are simply infections of the nail itself. Various types of fungal infections, known as onychomycosis (Figure 18.2), can create nails that are white, green, yellow, or black in colour. The nails also tend to show various stages of disintegration. Most occur on people who work with their hands immersed in water for long periods or work with various chemicals. Most nail infections will be more severe on one hand (the active hand) or will have one or two nails (usually the thumbnails) free of problems.

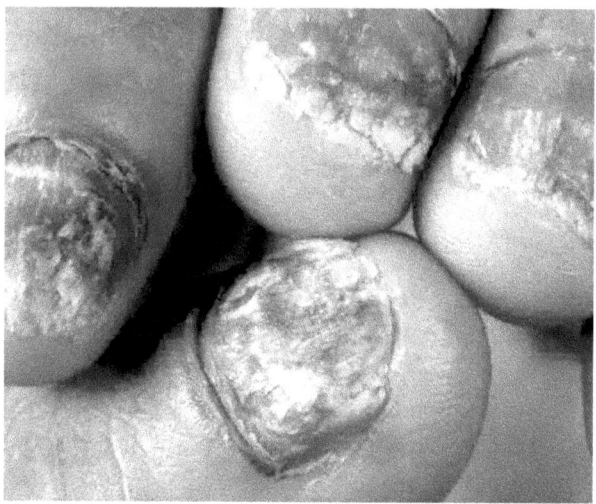

Figure 18.2. Onychomycosis.

Paronchia

Another non-chronic and quite common fungal infection is paronchia (Figure 18.3), which is inflammation of the nail fold, causing it to become red, hot, tender, and swollen. This, again, though it looks alarming, is actually a localised infection, caused by injury or irritation to the area around the nail. It is not a signal of a serious condition.

White spots on the nails

Leukonychia punctata (Figure 18.4) – as white spots on the nails are called – is by far the most common issue you'll spot on any set of nails. They are particularly widespread on teenagers living on late nights, pizzas, and energy drinks, on new, breastfeeding mothers, and on people who are run down after an illness. A few of these on a couple of nails are very often seen and nothing to

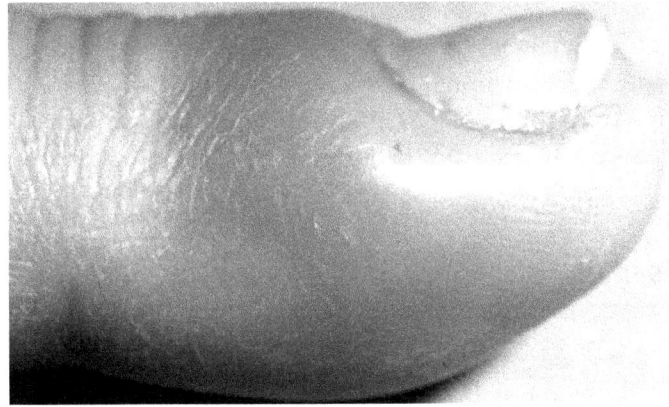

Figure 18.3. Paronchia.

worry about. Where all the nails have numerous white spots, this is a response to a depletion of minerals caused by exhaustion, stress, being run down, poor diet, or, in particular, excess consumption of refined sugars. The body compensates for any depletion by utilising the trace minerals from the nails and other non-essential

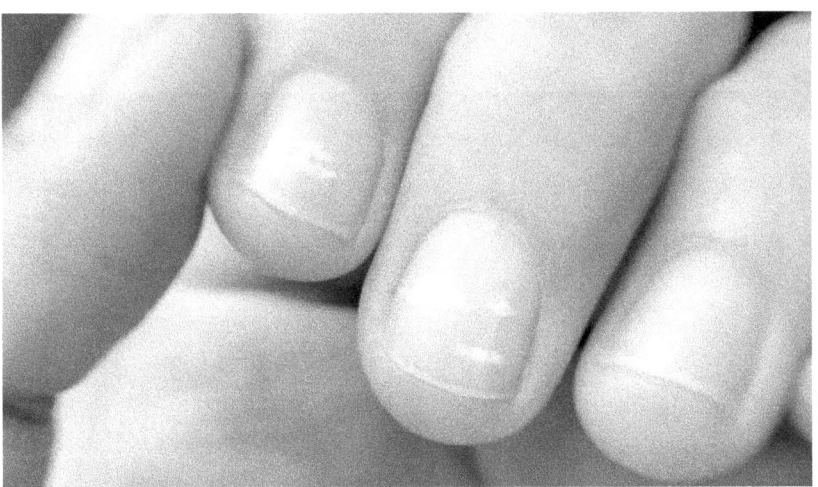

Figure 18.4. White spots on the nails.

tissues of the body, thereby diminishing its resources. The most common deficiencies are zinc, thiamine, copper, and calcium. If the cause is nutritional, reducing the intake of refined sugars and increasing the intake of zinc and other trace minerals should restore normality in a few months.

Beau's lines

Beau's lines (Figure 18.5) are common. They are horizontal depressions in the nail plate that run parallel to the lanula. They grow out as the nail grows. These arise from a sudden interruption of nail growth. The extent of the problem determines the width of the groove – wider and on all the nails in severe cases. It usually occurs after a severe illness and infection, such as pneumonia, myocardial infarction, or even emotional stress. One can determine when the illness occurred by looking at the location of the line. As nails take six months to grow out, if the line is halfway up the nail, the illness would have occurred three months previously. The interruption of nail growth may also occur after shock, malnutrition, and weight loss. Chemotherapy drugs also produce these lines.

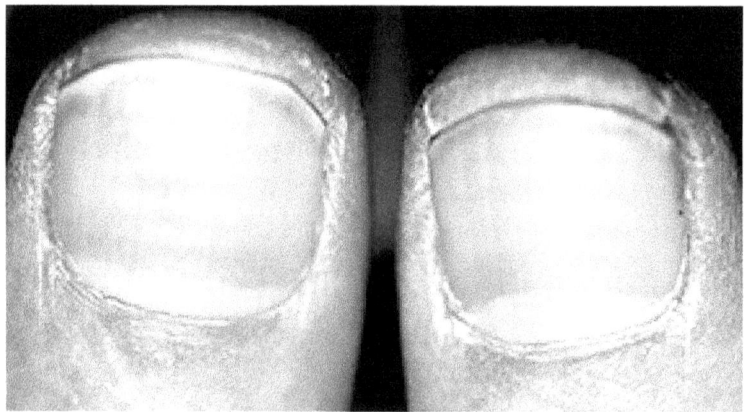

Figure 18.5. Beau's lines.

Vertical ridges on the nails

Fine vertical ridges tend to appear as we age, and if only on a few nails (the ring finger predominately) and not too deep, this is normal and of no consequence. However, if the ridges form deep grooves running up the length of all the nails, it is most likely a sign of gout, arthritis, or systemic sclerosis.

Mee's lines

Sometimes a single band of white appears on the nails, running from side to side across the width of the nail plate. These slowly move towards the fingertip as the nail grows. These are known as Mee's lines (Figure 18.6), and the width of the band varies according to the extent of the problem. This shows periods of time when the body has been under severe toxicity load, such as in heavy metal poisoning (arsenic, thallium, and selenium), renal dysfunction, chemotherapy, serious illness, or a period of time spent at high altitude mountaineering.

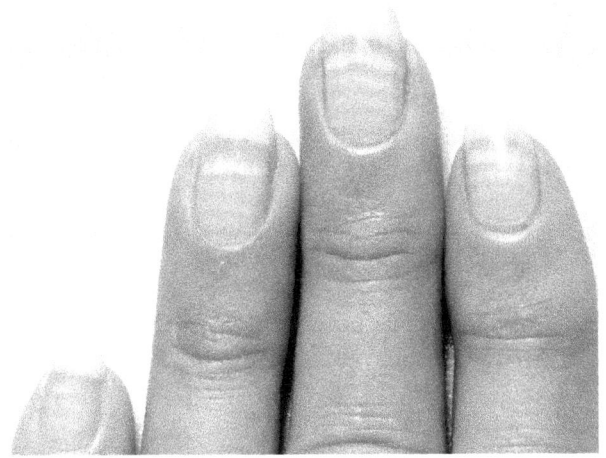

Figure 18.6. Mee's lines.

Thickening, breaking, and splitting nails

Nails that are slow-growing and very dry and brittle and crack or split vertically are deficient in vitamins A, biotin, and essential fatty acids. Eating disorders and chemotherapy will create chronic nail brittleness due to protein deficiency. Nails often become brittle in very old age due to decreasing ability to absorb nutrients.

Soft nails

Frequent exposure to water softens nails, which makes them highly susceptible to damage and infection. The nails are very absorbent (ten times more absorbent than skin), so water saturates the nail, especially after constant immersion. The water then diffuses back out, and this constant change in water content causes the cells to expand, contract, and soften. Where there has been no prolonged water exposure, soft, thin, pliable nails occur as a result of protein deficiency from a poor diet, which can be resolved by consuming protein-rich foods to build tissue, in addition to minerals and vitamins.

Splinter haemorrhage

Splinter haemorrhages are longitudinal streaks in the nails, brown-red in colour (Figure 18.7). They don't blanch when pressure is applied. These are caused by trauma, drugs, systemic diseases, and idiopathic conditions. Trauma is by far the most common cause in a situation where, for instance, the fingertips get trapped in a door. The far more serious issue of infective endocarditis should be suspected if accompanied by Osler's nodes or Janeway lesions (Chapter 19).

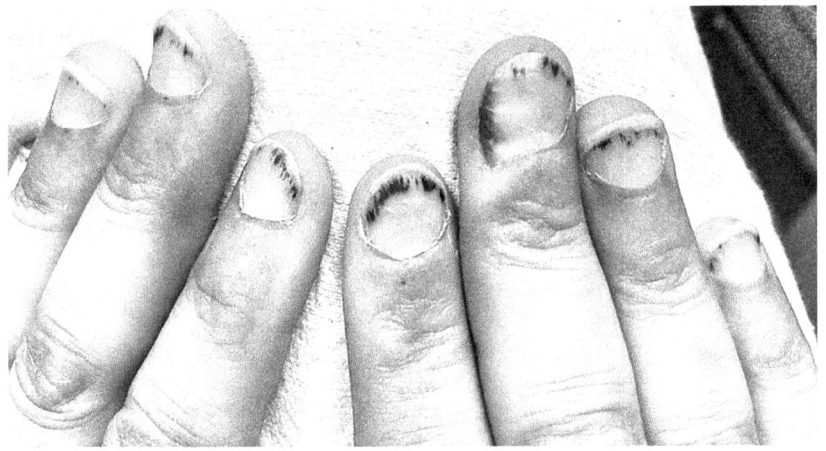

Figure 18.7. Splinter haemorrhages.

Terry's nails

Terry's nails (Figure 18.8) occur when the lanula extends to more than 75% of the nail, with most of the nail plate being thin; giving the nails a ground glass appearance. It usually occurs on all the nails. This is due to a decrease in blood supply and an increase in connective tissue in the nail bed. It occurs in states of bodily stress, such as very advanced age, liver diseases, (cirrhosis), chronic renal failure, congestive heart failure, diabetes, and malnutrition.

Missing nail moons

If there is no trace of the lanula on all the fingers and thumbs, it may be indicative of anaemia, low cellular oxygen, poor circulation, or malnutrition. A series of pale blue moons may be suggestive of diabetes mellitus.

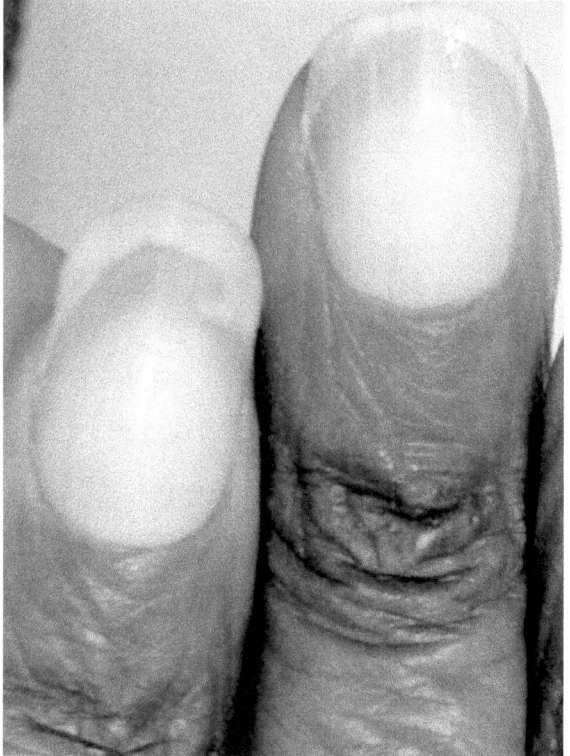

Figure 18.8. Terry's nails.

Nail colour

Nail chromonychia is defined as an abnormality of the nail plate colour not due to nail infection. It is vital to rule this out first and to make sure any colouration is not a result of external factors, such as exposure or dyes like henna, ink, chemicals, or nicotine on smoker's nails. Generally, fungal infections create a flaky deterioration in the nail itself, and one or two fingers will be clear of the issue. Chromanychia discolouration due to internal factors tends to be present on all nails, and the colour is stronger nearer the moons. Certain drugs, including minocycline, cancer chemotherapy agents, and anti- malarial drugs may cause discolouration.

Green nails

Green nails are caused by advanced emphysema, due to a severe lack of oxygen in the bloodstream.

Blue nails

Blue nails indicate constriction of blood supply. They may be present with cyanosis, which is an inability of the body to supply oxygenated red blood to the extremities, due to cardiac-related conditions. Blue nails may indicate iron deficiency (anaemia) or heart or circulatory conditions.

Yellow nails

Yellow nails (not caused by nicotine or other exposure) will tend to occur with nails that thicken and grow very slowly. The sides of the nail show an exaggerated convex shape and become claw-like; the lanula disappears, and all the nails have a faint yellow hue. It is most often seen in patients with jaundice, liver disease, chronic bronchiectasis or sinusitis, pleural effusions, internal malignancies, immunodeficiency syndromes, and rheumatoid arthritis.

White nails

White nails may be indicative of severe anaemia, vascular conditions, or oedema.

Purple nails

Purple nails are generally due to a deprivation of oxygen and circulatory problems.

Black/brown nails

Black or brown nails are very rare as indicators of medical conditions and usually indicate nail infection or trauma to the nail or nail bed. If occurring on all the nails, it's common where there has been excessive fluoride ingestion. Other conditions may also include diabetes mellitus, cardiovascular disease, or syphilis.

Lindsay's nails

Lindsay's nails (Figure 18.9) have a brown band across the top part of the nails from an increased pigment deposition. They are also called "half and half" nails, as the lower part of the nail is dull

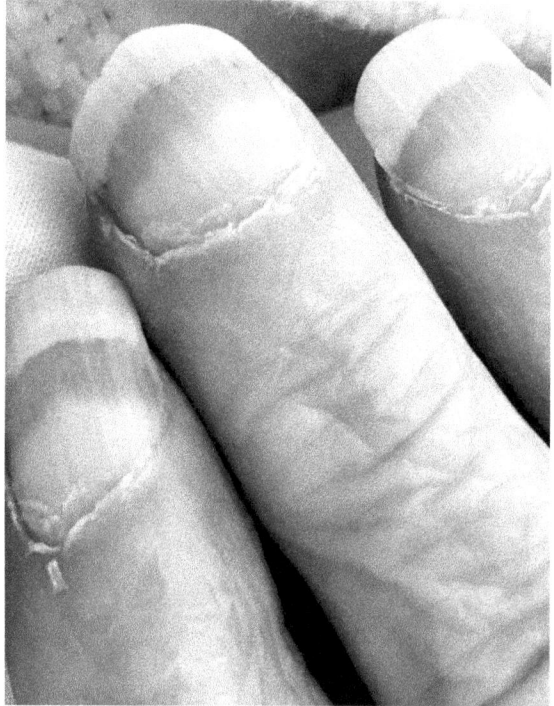

Figure 18.9. Lindsay's nails.

white and opaque, obscuring the lanula. This is associated with chronic renal disease, uraemia, as well as HIV and is also found in renal transplant patients on haemodialysis.

Other nail conditions

Koilonychia

Koilonychia (spoon nails) (Figure 18.10) is a condition marked by a concave, depressed lower part of the nail, which becomes thin and with a lift at the outer edges. The depression may even be deep enough hold a drop of water. The nail appears distorted in the way plastic warps when heated. The two most common conditions associated with spoon nails are iron deficiency (Plummer-Vinson syndrome) or poor absorption of iron; or, sometimes, protein deficiency, especially sulphur-containing amino acids.

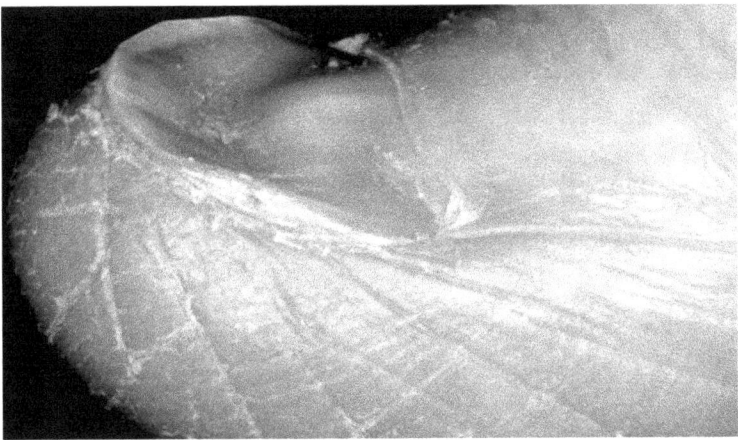

Figure 18.10. Spoon nails.

Pitting of the nails

Pitting nails (Figure 18.11) are tiny, punctuated depressions on the surface from loss of cells from the nail plate. Pits can vary in depth and in amount. This is almost always a sign of psoriasis, but may also be associated with reactive arthritis or alopecia areata (hair loss).

Digital clubbing

Clubbing (Figure 18.12) is a clinically descriptive term, referring to a bulbous uniform swelling of the fingertip so they resemble the rounded end of drumsticks and result in a swollen, convex curve of the nails. In all cases of clubbing a deficiency of oxygen is indicated, with deficiency in the haemoglobin content of the blood. Some form of serious illness is suspected, such as infective endocarditis, congenital heart disease, TB, chronic bronchitis, CPOD, empyema, lung abscess, and lung cancer.

Improving nail health

Primary treatment for nails in poor condition is based on restoring whole-body balance via the addition of elements or through elimination of toxins. Essential fatty acids are excellent to moisturise the nail bed, which increases nail flexibility, especially for thin and brittle nails. Minerals, such as silica, facilitate the absorption of calcium, which improves the strength of nails and helps to reduce nail breakage. Natural silica is found in nettle, horsetail, burdock root, and oat straw, which can be used in herbal teas. Nettle, prickly ash, and rue improve peripheral circulation and increase the size of moons, particularly if aerobic exercise is taken up. Foods rich in phosphorus help to maintain and repair tissues

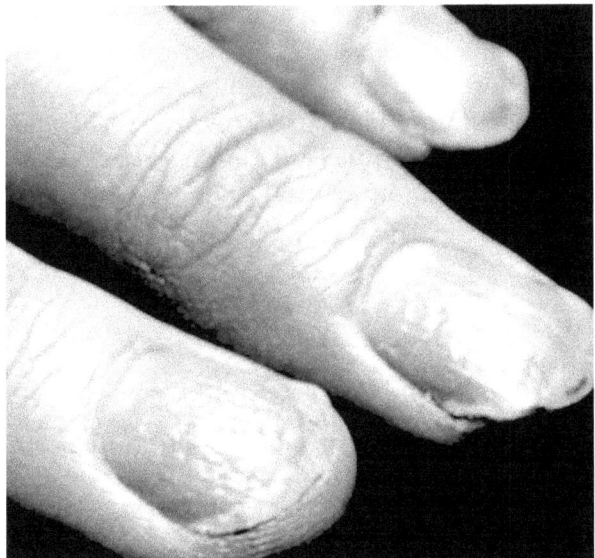

Figure 18.11. Nail pitting.

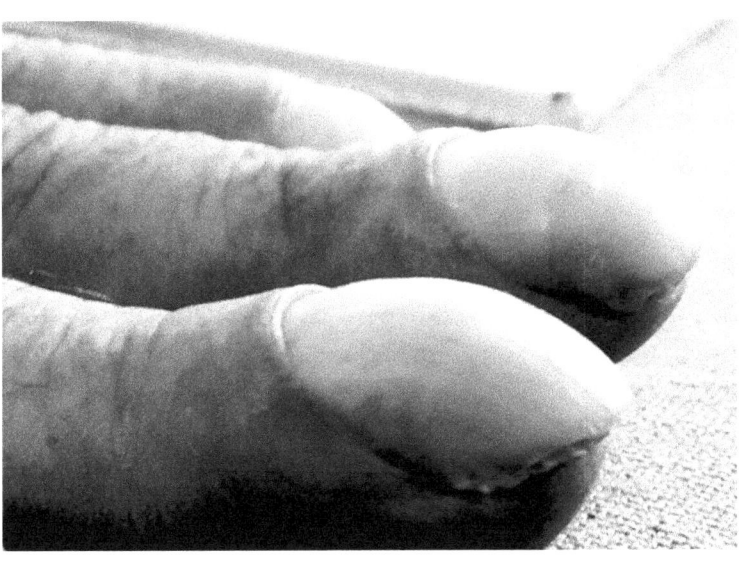

Figure 18.12. Digital clubbing.

and cells and aids in the growth and hardening of nails. Sulphur is an essential mineral that assists in the growth of nails and is an important constituent of keratin. Linseed, millet, yarrow, and comfrey are good nutritional sources to grow healthy nails, bones, and ligaments. Calcium, iron, and zinc from natural sources are essential for the formation of strong bones and nails.

Sources

Berman, K. (2014). *Brittle Nails.* https://s3.amazonaws.com/cafewell-content/adam012013/HIE%20Multimedia/2/9136.htm

Dugdale, D. C. (2013). *Capillary Nail Refill Test.* www.nlm.nih.gov/medlineplus/ency/article/003394.htm

Fawcett, S. Hart, T. M. Linford, S. & Stulberg, D. L. "Nail abnormalities: Clues to systemic disease." *American Family Physician,* Vol. 69, No. 6 (2004): 1417–1424.

Mash, B., Blitz, J., Kitshoff, D., & Naude, S. *South African Clinical Practitioners Manual* (Pretoria: Van Schaik, 2010).

Mendiratta, V., & Jain, A. "Nail dyschromias." *Indian Journal of Dermatology, Venereology and Leprology,* Vol. 77, No. 6 (2011): 652–658.

Wild, D. B. (2012). *The Skin, Tongue and Nails Speak* (Loveland, CO: Unique Perspective Press, 2012).

Williams, M. E. (2014). *Examining the Fingernails.* Charlottesville, VA: University of Virginia School of Medicine. https://med.virginia.edu/dom/wp-content/uploads/sites/210/2015/11/NailExamination.pdf

19

Common acute conditions

Hopefully, this book has given you a thorough understanding of the power of hand analysis as a diagnostic tool. Not only can you ascertain if a client has a higher statistical chance of developing a disease or condition, but you can also see where an issue may be just starting to emerge and also where a problem is present or acute. As stated at the beginning of this book, the hand is amazing for its capacity to indicate problems long before they become serious, and with complementary therapy, change of diet, and lifestyle, they can often be overcome without recourse to conventional medicine or drugs.

Following the methodology of this book, you can work your way through a progression of layers of how strong the evidence is of a medical condition. There may be a constitutional likelihood of illness seen through studying the hand shape, skin texture, and finger length; more likelihood may be found from statistical indications of finger and palm prints; yet firmer signals may be provided by the major and minor lines and skin ridges; and finally, firm evidence of a current and ongoing condition may be seen in hand tremors and in the fingernails.

A good benchmark for a medical palm diagnosis is seeing *three* signs of a condition. So, for instance, you may have a client with eight-whorl fingerprints, red dots on the water line, and a blue tinge to all the nails. These, taken together, indicate not only a likelihood, but an active and potentially serious heart condition. Despite this evidence, we must recognise that we are *not* medical specialists, and we can only urge our clients towards a more in-depth examination and quick follow-up when we see an issue. We must never diagnose – only gently push towards a more thorough diagnosis.

The following medical conditions are the most common issues that I have personally come across through 40 years of hand reading. Each of these is an acute, possibly life-threatening problem and needful of immediate medical attention. Even with little experience and perhaps just starting to utilise medical hand reading in your practice, if you see the indications mentioned below, it's vital that the client takes action and gets a formal follow up as soon as possible.

Common danger signs in the hands needing immediate medical attention

Severe anaemia

This is easily the issue you'll come across most often, particularly on menstruating females or those on any form of restricted diet. The indications are: white or very pale nails or spoon-shaped nails (koilonychia) that have a concave depression near the base. When stretched out, the inner palm's lines don't show as pink but remain white. The capillary nail refill test (where the nail is pressed till white) takes more than three seconds to refill with colour. The hands are cold and pale. The patient will report dizziness, lack of energy, shortness of breath, and lassitude.

Hyperthyroidism

This is the most common endocrine issue seen in the hands. This is when the thyroid gland produces low levels of hormone leading to many of the body's functions slowing down. This is indicated by lots of scratchy markings on the tip of the little fingers of both hands and markings on all fingertips; cold hands at room temperature; no moons, or very pale nails that make the moons invisible. The hands feel dry and doughy. This condition should be strongly flagged if there has been unusual weight gain, lethargy, and aching muscles, and if the client is a woman between the ages of 20 and 40 (this condition is 10 times more common in women than in men and is particularly prevalent in this age range). It is estimated that more than 5% of adults have this condition to some extent, and many go undiagnosed until symptoms become chronic.

Diabetes

Diabetes is very common and is often undiagnosed – up to 25% of sufferers in the United States have the condition and are unaware of it, according to a Center for Disease Control and Prevention report (*National Diabetes Statistics Report*). The signs in the hand are: water line ends by dropping down to near or onto the earth line; trigger finger; Terry's nails, or nails with missing moons or blue moons; brown or black nails not caused by infection; pins and needles in the hands; muscle wastage at the back of the hand, between index and thumb (Figure 19.1). This is accompanied by frequent urination, constant thirst, exhaustion, blurred vision, and very dry skin.

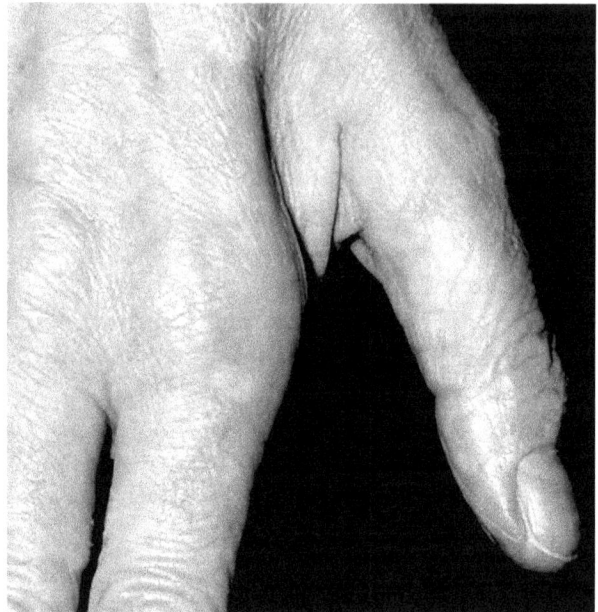

Figure 19.1. Muscle wastage at the back of the hand in diabetes.

Tripe palms

Tripe palms (palmar hyperkeratosis: Figure 19.2) describes a condition in which the skin of the palm becomes thick and velvety-white, with pronounced folds in the lines of the hand. This is immediately obvious: the skin resembles boiled tripe. This is an ominous sign, as it usually signals cancer (up to 95% of tripe palms indicate cancer of some form). The patient needs to be referred to a cancer clinic the same day, if at all possible. If only the palms are involved, it's most probably lung cancer. If tripe palms are accompanied by acanthosis nigricans (similar thick, velvety skin in the armpits, groin, and neck), the underlying malignancy is most commonly stomach (35%) or lung (11%) cancer.

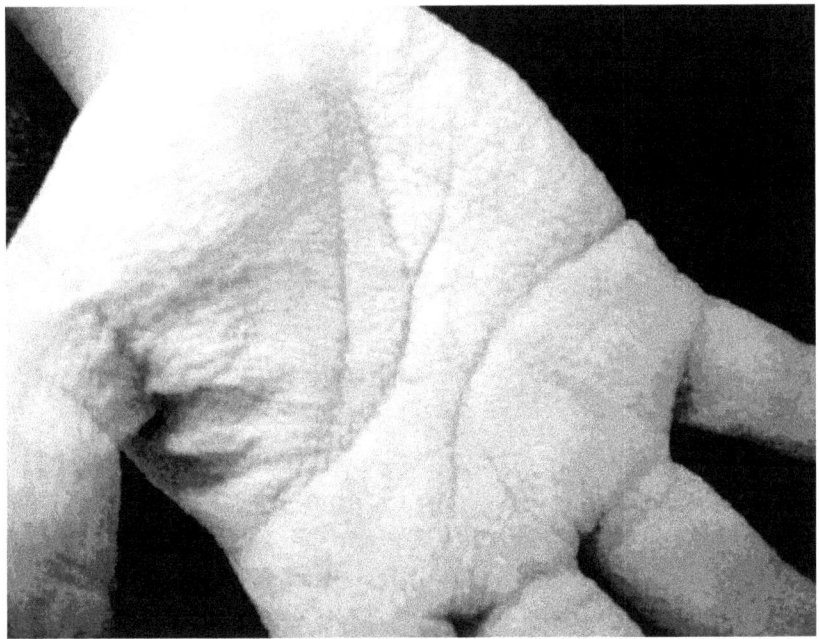

Figure 19.2. Tripe palms.

Heart conditions

Obviously, any heart condition is a serious issue. Palm predispositions include a fire hand, a large number of fingertip whorls, a highly placed axial triradius, and a single transverse crease line. Water line features include a line that is very weak and chained for much of its course, a hard nodule beneath the ring finger, red dots, break-up of skin ridges beneath the ring digit, and a complete crossing water line. Signs of an active condition include blue, black, or white nails (not caused by chemical contamination or nail infection). Clubbed fingertips alone should always be seen as a sign of a serious condition and medical attention sought quickly. The capillary nail refill test is a good measure of circulation issues. If there are indicators of heart condition,

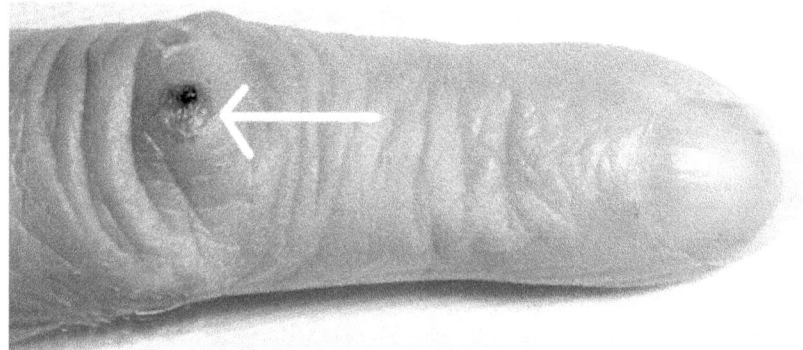

Figure 19.3.   Osler's nodes.

another sign of serious problems (not previously mentioned) are: Osler's nodes (Figure 19.3) and Janeway lesions (Figure 19.4). Osler's nodes are typically painful red 1–10 mm nodules on the fingers, and Janeway lesions are pain-free irregular-shaped markings on the palms. These can be a sign of bacterial endocarditis (inflammation of the inside lining of the heart), which is a

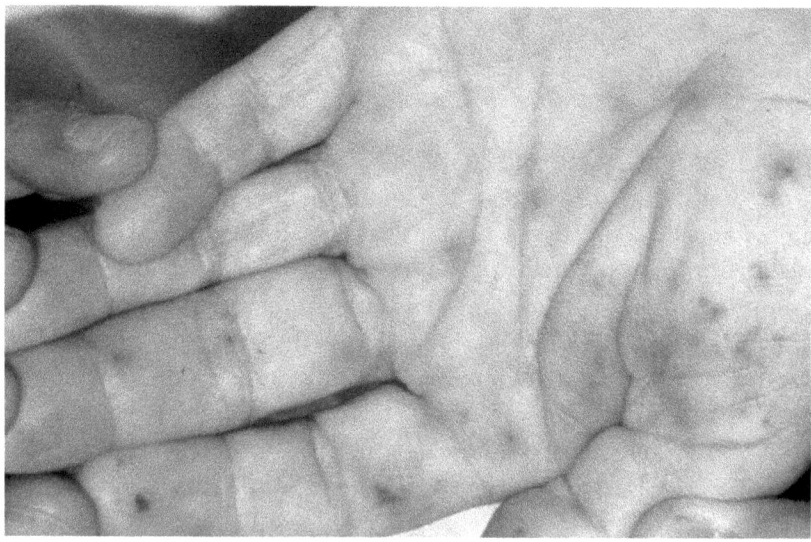

Figure 19.4.   Janeway lesions.

dangerous condition. The most common symptoms of endocarditis are fever, chills and sweating, fatigue, loss of appetite, and muscle aches and pains.

Arthritis

The hands are often the first part of the body to signal the beginning of arthritis. A slight stiffening of the fingers and a slightly painful thumb joint are the earliest indications. There are usually signs of veiling (a dense cluster of very fine lines) on the percussion (opposite side to the thumb) edge of the palm, with some skin ridge break-up in the same area. The finger knuckles may swell slightly, and all the nails begin to show pronounced vertical ridges. The nails often become slightly yellowish, and growth becomes very slow. An elimination diet to clean the system of acidity is highly recommended at the first suggestion of arthritis, and a nutritional therapist should be consulted.

Sources

Centers for Disease Control and Prevention (U.S.). *National Diabetes Statistics Report: Estimates of Diabetes and Its Burden in the United States Updated and Reviewed: 29 November, 2023* (Washington, DC: CDC).
Ellenberg, M. "Diabetic Neuropathy of the Upper Extremities." *Journal of the Mount Sinai Hospital*, Vol. 35, No. 2 (1968): 131–148.
Eswaraiah, G., & Bali, S ."Palmar flexion creases and dermatoglyphics among diabetic patients." *American Journal of Physical Anthropology*, Vol. 47, No. 1 (1977): 11–13.
Rashad, M. "Dermatoglyphic traits in patients with cardiovascular disorders". *American Journal of Physical Anthropology*, Vol. 42, No. 2 (1975): 281–283.
Sayan, O. R., & Carter, W. A. "Endocarditis (Dermatologic signs and symptoms)." In: J. G. Adams (Ed.), *Emergency Medicine, Second Edition* (Philadelphia, PA: Elsevier, 2013).

APPENDIX

Further reading

Jaquin, N. *The Hand Speaks* (London: Faber, 1942).
Manning, J. *The Finger Book* (London: Faber & Faber, 2009).
Scheimann, E., & Altman, N. *Medical Palmistry: A Doctor's Guide to Better Health Through Palmistry* (Wellingborough: Aquarian Press, 1989).
Wild, D. B. (2012). *The Skin, Tongue and Nails Speak* (Loveland, CO: Unique Perspective Press).
PubMed (https://pubmed.ncbi.nlm.nih.gov) has thousands of scientific papers linking palm markings to health issues. To find medical palmistry research papers on the site, you need to type in scientific names for hand features. For instance, for information on the ring finger length you will need to type: "2D4D ratio", and to find out about a print pattern you will need to type the specific type of print, i.e.: "simple arch dermatoglyphics".

Recommended websites

Unfortunately 90% of palmistry websites are a mess of mumbo-jumbo and predictive twaddle. A few that are worth visiting, with real insights and useful information, are the following:

www.handreading.nz
www.handanalysis.co.uk
www.handreadingbyfelicity.co.uk
www.handresearch.com

My own website is:

johnnyfincham.com

INDEX

Aarskog-Scott syndrome, 93
acanthosis nigricans, 170
active hand, 8, 32, 73, 74, 78, 81, 89, 104, 106, 117, 153
acute conditions, 167–173
air element, 17
air hand(s), 12, 19
air line(s), 19, 64, 65, 79, 112, 113
   bent, 88–89
   breaks in, 89–91
   clarity of, 85–87
   curved, 88, 137
   double, 137
   and earth line:
     joined, 80
     separate, 81
   frazzled, 86
   island on, 86, 87, 137
     large, 87
   length of, 82–83
   long, 83
   major, 79–93
   messy beginning of, 81
   nature of, 79
   path of, 87–89
   second, 136
   short, 82, 134
   Sydney, 84
   in two sections, 91
   very bent, 88
   after yoga training, 90
air palm, 19, 134

allergy line, 119, 130–131
   dominant, 120
Alter, Milton, 54
Altman, Nathaniel, 61
anaemia, 85, 159, 161, 168
Apollo line, 128
arch, 48
   simple, 44, 46–47, 53, 55
   tented, 44, 47–48, 56, 134
Aristotle, 2
art, 11
arthritis, 38, 42, 55, 59, 133, 157, 161, 164, 173
astrology, 11
axial triradius, 57, 85, 93, 171
   normal and raised, 58

bacterial endocarditis, 172
basal phalanges, large, 39
Beau's lines, 156
behavioural patterns, 7
Bell, Charles, 2
Bhanu, V., 85
Bim, M. A., 35
black nails, 162, 169, 171
blood disorders, 6
blue moons, 159, 169
blue nails, 161, 171
brain and hand development, link between, 3
brain motor and nerve, proportion of allocation in body, 4

Brandon-Jones, David, 30
breast cancer, 15, 41, 55, 59–60
broken earth lines, 71
brown nails, 162
Buddhist cosmology, 11

capillary nail refill test, 153, 168, 171
cerebellar tremor, 149
cholesterol, high, 14, 100
clubbed fingertips, 171
clubbing, digital, 2, 164
coeliac disease, 146
complementary medicine/therapy, 2, 6
composite fingerprint, 56
composite loop, 51–52, 56, 57
constipation, 14, 55, 124
constitutional types, 11–20
constitutions, basic, 11
control, willpower, resources, 30
cortex, motor and sensory, portion devoted to palms, 3
Cummins, H., 43
cuticle, 151, 152

dermal ridge erosion, 144–145
dermatoglyphics, 43, 53, 54–58
design, 11
destiny line, 108
diagnostic tool, hand as, 7
diabetes, 42, 104, 133, 159, 162, 169
  muscle wastage at back of hand in, 170
digital clubbing, 2, 164, 165
digits, floppy, 38
disease, predispositions to, 8
dominant hand, as active hand, 8
dots along water line, 98
Down's syndrome, 3, 5

earth element, 13–14
earth hand(s), 12, 14, 16
earth line(s), 14, 64, 65, 104, 108, 115, 122, 130, 135, 136, 145, 146, 147, 169
  and air line:
    joined, 80
    separate, 81
  broken, 71–72
    no overlap, 73
    with overlap, 72
  fire line beginning on, 116
  fire line replacing section of, 117
  island on, 74, 75
  major, 67–78
  missing base of, 73–75
  narrow sweep to, 78
  nature of, 67
  nibbled edges on, 76
  short, weak, 69
  strong, 68
  sweep of, 76–78
  weak, 131, 138
  wide sweep to, 77
earth palms, 12
Edwards syndrome, 55
elemental hand shapes, 12
elements, four: fire, water, earth, and air, 11
emotional idealism, 102
empyema, 2
endocarditis, 173
  bacterial, 172
  infective, 158, 164
endocrine system, 138–140
epidermal ridges, 43, 58

fate line, 108
finger(s), 36–42
  flexible, 38
  index, 26, 32, 40, 86, 94, 100, 102, 136, 148
  middle, 65, 80, 86, 94, 100, 107, 108, 109
  ring, 40, 41, 42, 86, 96, 106, 139, 157, 171
  testing for flexibility, 37
  trigger, 42
finger flexibility, 37–38
finger length, 40, 167
finger-length configurations, as indicators, 3
finger phalanges, 39–40
fingerprint(s), 1, 3, 21, 26, 54, 55, 59, 62, 93, 143, 167
  composite, 56
  eight-whorl, 168
  patterns, 43–53
  whorl, 44
fingerprint formations, 21
fingerprint patterns, 3, 43, 54–58
  five, 44
fingertips, 49, 93, 96, 139, 140, 158, 169

clubbed, 171
endocrine system markers on, 138
fingertip whorls, 171
Finley, B., 42
fire element, 16
fire hand(s), 12, 17, 51, 171
fire line(s), 17, 64, 65, 108, 108–118
   appearing halfway, 112–113
   beginning on earth line, 116
   complete crossing, 113, 114
   fast developing, 117–118
   fractured, 138
   island in, 111
   lack of, 109–111
   nature of, 108
   palm lacking, 110
   replacing section of earth line, 116–117
   scratchy, striated, 114–115
fire palm(s), 12, 16, 52
Fitzherbert, Andrew, 83
flexibility, finger, 37, 37–38
floppy digits, 38
fungal infections, 153–159, 154

Galton, Francis, 43
Girdle of Venus line, 121
green nails, 161, 298
gut biota, 70

haemorrhages, splinter, 158, 159
hand(s):
   active, 8
   air, 12
   changed, 9
   child's, at 7-month intervals, 10
   cold, 95, 169
   danger signs in, 168
   during difficulties, 110, 134
   as diagnostic tool, 2, 7
   earth, 12, 14
   elemental nature of, 11
   fire, 12
   green, 161
   minor lines of, 7
   muscle wastage at back of, in diabetes, 170
   passive, 8
   pins and needles in, 169
   and underlying health problem, 6
   water, 12

hand analysis, power of, as diagnostic tool, 167
hand development, and brain development, link between, 3
handprints, taking, 21–24
hand shapes, 19, 62, 167
   elemental, 12
   fundamental, four, 11
hand tremors, 167
   involuntary, 148–150
Hashemian, S. S., 41, 42
head line, 4
health line, 123
heart condition, 168, 171
heart line, 4
hepatica, 123
Hindu cosmology, 11
Hippocrates, 1, 2
hyperthyroidism, 169
immune-system disorders, 15, 55
index finger, 26, 32, 40, 86, 94, 100, 102, 136, 139, 148
index finger length and ring finger length, 40–42
infective endocarditis, 158, 164
intensity line, 120, 129–130, 138
island(s):
   air line, 86
   in fire line, 111
   on air line, 137
   in vagus nerve line, 125

Janeway lesions, 158, 172
Jaquin, Noel, 61, 143, 144

Kasielska-Trojan, A., 41, 42
keratin, 151, 152, 166
Klinefelter syndrome, 56, 93
koilonychia, 163, 168
kundalini meditation course, 127

lanula, 152, 156, 159, 161, 163
LetsGetChecked, 1
leukonychia punctata, 154
lifeline, 67, 71
Lindsay's nails, 162
line(s):
   air: *see* air line(s)
   earth: *see* earth line(s)
   fire: *see* fire line(s)
   length of, 65

line(s) (*continued*)
  major: *see* major line(s)
    beginnings and ends of, 61, 62, 65, 84, 108, 113, 119, 136
  minor, 119–132
  water: *see* water line(s)
line changes, 63
little finger, 4, 36, 50, 65, 82, 86, 93, 94, 123, 135, 139, 151
liver line, 123
liver tremor, 149
loop(s), 49–51, 53, 55
  composite, 51–52
  radial, 56
  ulnar, 49–50
lordosis, 15

major line(s), 64, 65, 71, 84, 102, 108, 113, 119
  beginning points, 66
  beginnings and ends of, 61, 62, 65, 84, 108, 113, 119, 136
  stress markings on, 136–137
Manning, John, 3
medical palm diagnosis, 167
medical palm reading/palmistry, 4, 21
medicine, complementary, 6
Mee's lines, 157
mental health, crucial and proven aspect of physical health, 2
mercury line, 123
middle finger, 19, 26, 36, 38, 64, 65, 80, 82, 86, 94, 100, 107–109, 113, 139
Midlo, C., 43, 59, 60
minor lines:
  major points of, 119–120
  super strong, 138
mirage line, 120, 121, 138
  fragmented, 122
mixed palm, 20
mysticism, 15

nail(s)/fingernail(s):
  black, 162, 169, 171
  blue, 161, 171
  brown, 162
  cross section of, 152
  green, 161
  health check using, 153
  Lindsay's, 162
  pale, 168, 169
  pitting, 164
  purple, 161
  soft, 158
  splitting, 158
  spoon-shaped, 163, 168
  Terry's, 159, 160, 169
  vertical ridges on, 157
  white, 161, 171
  white spots on, 154, 155
  yellow, 161
nail bed, 151, 152, 153, 159, 162, 164
nail brittleness, 158
nail chromonychia, 160–163
nail moons, 152
  missing, 159
nail pitting, 165
nail plate, 152, 156, 157, 159, 164
  colour, 160
Neptune line, 121
nerve and brain motor, proportion of allocation in body, 4
nervous tremor, 150
neurology, 2
Noonan syndrome, 93

ocean floor, 46–47
onychomycosis, 153, 154
Osler's nodes, 158, 172
osteoarthritis, 38, 41

paganism, 11
pale nails, 168, 169
palm(s):
  and disease, links between, 3
  composite print on, 57
  earth, 12
  fire, 12
  lines and markings on, changes in, 9
  no fire line, 110
  reflection of state of health, 1
  tripe, 170
  undefined, 12, 19
  water, 12
palmar crease, single transverse, 4, 91–93
palmar hyperkeratosis, 170
palmar skin:
  ridges in, 26
  thin, silky, 27
  ultra-coarse, 28

palm diagnosis, medical, 4, 119, 167
palmistry, 4, 7, 8, 11, 30, 33, 40, 44, 71,
    108, 128, 131
palm line(s):
    basic principles of, 64–65
    major, 61–66, 84, 108, 113, 119, 136
palm prints, 27, 43, 167
    example, 24
    method, 22
palm reading:
    medical, 21
    not qualified to diagnose, 6
Paracelsus, 2
Parkinson disease, 149
Parkinson's tremor, 148
paronchia, 154, 155
passive hand, 8, 40, 71, 73, 78, 80, 81,
    84, 88, 89, 104, 106, 109
Patau syndrome, 55, 93
pharmaceutical drugs, 6
pitting nails, 164
Plummer-Vinson syndrome, 163
print, whorl, 45, 55
prostate problems, 15
purple nails, 161

radial loop(s), 50–51, 56
rheumatoid arthritis, 38, 42, 55, 59, 161
ring finger, 82, 86, 96, 106, 139, 157,
    171
    and index finger length, 40–42
    island on water line beneath, 97
    long, 41
Ring of Saturn line, 121

Saturn line, 108
Schaumann, B., 54, 58–60
Schienmann, Eugene, 61
self-diagnosis, 1
Shamai-Lubovitz, O., 60
shiatsu, 129
silk skin, 27–28
silky skin, 134
simian line, 4
simple arch, 44, 46, 47, 53, 55
Singh, P. K., 59
single transverse palmar crease, 4,
    91–93
skin:
    coarse, 26, 28
    thin, 27

skin ridge(s):
    breaking up of, 143–147
    broken, 21, 144
skin ridge patterns, 21
skin surface and nervous system, 25
skin texture, 1, 25, 26, 62, 167
splinter haemorrhage(s), 158, 159
spoon nails, 163, 168
stomach and digestive issues, 14
stress, 133–142
    long-term, 133
    strategies to reduce, 140–142
stress lines:
    opposite Venus mount, 136
    within Venus mount, 135
stress markers, 134–136
string of pearls, 143–147
sublimation line, 120, 128
    on shiatsu practitioner's hand, 129
Suff, Rachel, 111
sun, line of, 128
Sydney air line, 84
Sydney lines, 83–85

tented arch, 44, 47, 48, 56, 134
Terry, R. D., 159, 160, 169
Terry's nails, 159, 160, 169
thenar eminence, 33–35
thumb, 23, 30–35, 39, 42, 49, 50, 56, 65,
    123, 148, 169, 173
    wide-spaced, 33
thumb angle, 32
thumb ball, 30, 31, 67, 76, 77, 87
thumbnails, 151, 153
thyroid tremor, 150
toxic tremor, 149
traditional Chinese Medicine, 7, 128
transverse palmar crease, single, 91–93
tremor:
    cerebellar, 149
    liver, 149
    nervous, 150
    Parkinson's, 148
    thyroid, 150
    toxic, 149
trigger finger, 42
tripe palms, 170, 171
triradius:
    axial, 57, 58, 85, 93, 171
    raised, 57
Turner's syndrome, 55, 56

ulnar loop, 50
  right-hand index-finger, 49
ultra-coarse skin, 28
undefined palms, 12

vagus nerve line, 120, 123–127, 138
  island in, 125
  before kundalini meditation course, 127
Venus mount, 23, 33–35, 39, 56, 67, 129, 145
  stress lines opposite, 136
  stress lines within, 135
via lascivia, 130
vortex, 44

water element, 14
water hand, 12, 14, 16, 51
water line(s), 16, 64, 65, 94–107, 109, 112, 121, 128, 132, 168, 169, 171
  broken, 106
  complete crossing, 101–102
  crossing lines on, 97
  curved, 98
  deep, strong, 96
  with dots along its length, 98
  end of, dropped, 104, 105
  fractured, 106
  with idealistic ending, 103
  length of, 100
  long, 101
  low-set, 104, 105
  nature of, 94–95
  poor, 107
  poor-quality, 95, 96
  quality of, 95–98
  scratchy, 96
  short, 100
  straight, 99
  strong, clear, 96, 98
  trajectory of, 98–99
  weak, poor-quality, 95
water palm, 12, 16
white nails, 161, 171
whorl(s), 44, 45, 55
whorl prints, 44, 45, 55
wide-spaced thumb, 33
Wolff, Charlotte, 3
Wolf-Hirschhorn Syndrome, 93

yellow nails, 161

www.ingramcontent.com/pod-product-compliance
Ingram Content Group UK Ltd.
Pitfield, Milton Keynes, MK11 3LW, UK
UKHW021149220525
458809UK00005B/10